T0201357

Psychiatry Algorithms for Primary Care

Psychiatry Algorithms for Primary Care

GAUTAM GULATI
MBBS MD FRCPsych FRCPI PGDipLATHE (Oxon) FHEA
University of Limerick,
Ireland

WALTER CULLEN
MB BCh BAO DCH DObs MD MICGP MRCGP
GradDipUTL
University College Dublin,
Ireland

BRENDAN KELLY
MB BCh BAO MA MSc MA MD PhD DGov PhD MA (*jure
officii*) MCPsychI FRCPsych FRCPI FTCD
Trinity College Dublin,
Ireland

WILEY Blackwell

This edition first published 2021
© 2021 John Wiley & Sons Ltd

The right of Gautam Gulati, Walter Cullen, and Brendan Kelly to be identified as the authors of this work has been asserted in accordance with law.

Registered Office
John Wiley & Sons, Inc., 111 River Street, Hoboken, NJ 07030, USA
John Wiley & Sons Ltd, The Atrium, Southern Gate, Chichester, West Sussex, PO19 8SQ, UK

Editorial Office
9600 Garsington Road, Oxford, OX4 2DQ, UK

For details of our global editorial offices, customer services, and more information about Wiley products visit us at www.wiley.com.

Wiley also publishes its books in a variety of electronic formats and by print-on-demand. Some content that appears in standard print versions of this book may not be available in other formats.

Library of Congress Cataloging-in-Publication Data
Names: Gulati, Gautam, 1979– author. | Cullen, Walter, author. | Kelly,
    Brendan (Brendan D.), author.
Title: Psychiatry algorithms for primary care / Gautam Gulati, Walter
    Cullen, Brendan Kelly.
Description: First edition. | Hoboken, NJ : Wiley-Blackwell, 2021. |
    Includes bibliographical references and index.
Identifiers: LCCN 2020026511 (print) | LCCN 2020026512 (ebook) | ISBN
    9781119653561 (paperback) | ISBN 9781119653660 (adobe pdf) | ISBN
    9781119653677 (epub)
Subjects: MESH: Mental Disorders–diagnosis | Mental Disorders–therapy |
    Primary Health Care–methods | Clinical Decision-Making–methods
Classification: LCC RC454 (print) | LCC RC454 (ebook) | NLM WM 141 | DDC
    616.89–dc23
LC record available at https://lccn.loc.gov/2020026511
LC ebook record available at https://lccn.loc.gov/2020026512

Cover Design: Wiley

Set in 10/12pt STIX Two Text by SPi Global, Pondicherry, India

Printed and bound in Singapore by Markono Print Media Pte Ltd

10 9 8 7 6 5 4 3 2 1

To our families…

Contents

Part 4   Complex Scenarios   83

Part 5   Special Considerations in Prescribing   95

Part 6   Appendices   107

Part 7   Self-Assessment   123

Foreword

Patients commonly present mental health problems in primary care, but general practitioners and other primary health care professionals are often uncertain how best to diagnose and manage them. We are aware that presentations of mental illness are seldom straightforward, and we can often find it confusing to unravel the psychological dimensions of physical symptoms. Many of us are worried about the dangers of getting a diagnosis wrong: whether, on the one hand, we will unnecessarily or harmfully label people as mentally unwell when they are experiencing normal responses to the difficulties of daily life; or, on the other hand, whether we will fail to identify potentially serious problems such as schizophrenia or psychotic depression. And the crucial business of assessing clinical risk, especially with regard to suicidality, is frequently noted as a major concern amongst family doctors worldwide.

Fortunately, help is at hand.

Written by three senior and well-respected Irish clinical academics, with expertise in psychiatry and primary care, *Psychiatry Algorithms for Primary Care* addresses the wide variety of mental health problems commonly encountered in primary care. Starting with the essentials of history taking and mental state examination, the authors take us through the major psychiatric diagnoses before focusing helpfully not only on common presentations, such as insomnia, unexplained physical symptoms, and fatigue, but also on complex presentations such as self-harm, suicide, and aggression.

The book is specifically intended to assist the busy general practitioner who needs information and clinical advice delivered in a concise and accessible format. For each of the topics under discussion we are provided with pertinent, succinct, pragmatic algorithms setting out key facts and key actions, which cover what to say as well as what to do. There is clear guidance on what we general practitioners can reasonably be expected to do ourselves, and on the points at which we should consider involving our specialist colleagues.

This book is an invaluable aide-memoire for experienced general practitioners, as well as a highly relevant guide for general practitioners in training. The authors have deliberately – and successfully – designed it for use in real-time clinical encounters, when immediate support is needed.

I will be keeping a copy in my consulting room!

Christopher Dowrick BA MSc MD CQSW FRCGP
Professor of Primary Medical Care, University of Liverpool, UK
Chair, World Organization of Family Doctors Working Party on
Mental Health

Acknowledgements

We would like to thank the following colleagues for their assistance and contribution to this book:

Dr Vishnu Pradeep, Saint John of God Hospital, Dublin

Dr Kevin Lally, University of Limerick

Dr Valerie Ní Mhurchú, University College Cork

Dr Muireann O'Donnell, University Hospital Limerick

Dr Mohd Faisal, University of Limerick

Dr Nia Clendennen, UCD School of Medicine

Dr Barry O'Donnell, UCD School of Medicine

Dr Noreen Moloney, University of Limerick

Dr Elizabeth Fistein, Department of Public Health and Primary Care, University of Cambridge

Dr Darius Whelan, School of Law, University College Cork

Author Profiles

Gautam Gulati is Adjunct Associate Clinical Professor at the Graduate Entry Medical School at the University of Limerick and Consultant Forensic and General Psychiatrist. In addition to his medical degree (MBBS), he holds a Doctor of Medicine (MD) degree from the University of Limerick. He completed Higher Training in Forensic Psychiatry at Oxford and formerly worked at Oxford as Consultant Forensic Psychiatrist and Honorary Senior Clinical Lecturer. He has authored a well-read textbook on psychiatry and a number of peer-reviewed publications in national and international journals. He has taught at several universities including the University of Oxford, University College Cork, NUI Galway, and the University of Limerick. He is a Fellow of the Royal College of Psychiatrists (UK) and Fellow of the Royal College of Physicians of Ireland. He is Chair of the Faculty of Forensic Psychiatry at the College of Psychiatrists of Ireland and Convenor of the Diploma in Clinical Psychiatry Examination at the Royal College of Physicians of Ireland.

Walter Cullen is Professor of Urban General Practice at the School of Medicine in University College Dublin, Ireland. A practising GP since 1998, he works as a GP in Dublin's north inner city. He is a member of the Royal College of General Practitioners and Irish College of General Practitioners and was awarded an MD degree in 2005. His research focuses on the care of patients with mental health and substance-use disorders in primary care and has resulted in 200 peer-reviewed publications and two book chapters. He is Head of Subject (General Practice) at UCD and previously was Foundation Professor of General Practice at the University of Limerick.

Brendan D. Kelly is Professor of Psychiatry at Trinity College Dublin, Consultant Psychiatrist at Tallaght University Hospital, Dublin, and Visiting Full Professor at University College Dublin. In addition to his medical degree (MB BCh BAO), he holds master's degrees in epidemiology (MSc), healthcare management (MA), and Buddhist studies (MA), and an MA (*jure officii*) from Trinity College Dublin; and doctorates in medicine (MD), history (PhD), governance (DGov), and law (PhD). He has authored and co-authored over 250 publications in peer-reviewed journals, over 500 non-peer-reviewed publications, 14 book chapters and contributions, and 11 books (eight as sole author). His recent books include *Hearing Voices: The History of Psychiatry in Ireland* (2016), *Mental Illness, Human Rights and the Law* (2016), and *The Doctor Who Sat for a Year* (2019). He is a Fellow of the Royal College of Psychiatrists, the Royal College of Physicians of Ireland, and Trinity College Dublin. In 2017 he became Editor-in-Chief of the *International Journal of Law and Psychiatry*.

PART 1

Introduction

CHAPTER 1

How to Use This Book

One person in four will develop a mental illness at some point in life. The vast majority will suffer from mild to moderate depression, anxiety, or substance misuse. As a result, most mental healthcare is delivered in general practice. That is why we wrote this book: a book of psychiatry algorithms for general practice.

Our book is designed as a practical guide to psychiatric assessment and mental health care in day-to-day general practice. It is not a substitute for a medical degree, for continuing medical education, or for the systematic syntheses of evidence published by the National Institute for Health and Care Excellence (NICE). Instead, our book is aimed at informing rapid clinical decisions in busy surgeries and clinics.

With backgrounds in general practice and psychiatry, we recognise the need for guidance about both the mental health problems that are commonly seen in general practice and the problems that are rarely seen and are therefore more unfamiliar. So, this book is intended to assist in both of these situations, when rapid assessment and a treatment decision are needed for problems both familiar and unfamiliar.

The opening chapters of the book cover brief history taking in general practice and the rapid mental state examination, with an emphasis on what is achievable in busy clinical settings. Often, information emerges in a haphazard fashion during the course of a complex consultation; we suggest that this reminder of key headings for both the psychiatric history and the mental state examination can help identify and address gaps in the information provided.

Psychiatry Algorithms for Primary Care, First Edition. Gautam Gulati, Walter Cullen, and Brendan Kelly.
© 2021 John Wiley & Sons Ltd. Published 2021 by John Wiley & Sons Ltd.

These opening sections are followed by chapters devoted to specific psychiatric illnesses including anxiety disorders, obsessive compulsive disorder, depression, bipolar affective disorder, post-traumatic stress disorder, alcohol and substance misuse, psychosis (especially schizophrenia), eating disorders, delirium, dementia, personality disorders, autism spectrum disorder, and attention deficit hyperactivity disorder.

Not all patients present with a ready diagnosis, so the following chapters explore common complaints that can mask or suggest psychological or psychiatric disorders, such as insomnia, unexplained somatic symptoms, and fatigue ('tired all the time'). More complex scenarios are considered next, including self-harm, suicide, aggression, and referrals for involuntary care for severe mental disorder. These situations are always challenging.

Finally, we outline special considerations to be taken into account in the contexts of children, intellectual disability, the elderly, and pregnancy. The book's appendices cover commonly prescribed psychotropics, physical examination and investigations for people with severe mental illness, and MCQs for self-assessment.

Overall, this book aims to:

- provide a reminder of the essentials of psychiatric history-taking and mental state examination;
- present a compendium of pragmatic, usable algorithms for decision-making around psychiatric illness in general practice; and
- assist general practitioners and their teams in the delivery of high-quality, evidence-based, person-centred mental health care.

Disclaimer

This book is intended as general guidance only and does not in any way represent medical or legal advice for individual persons. Readers are advised to use their own academic and clinical knowledge when taking clinical decisions. While every effort has been made to ensure the accuracy of the information and material contained in this book, it is still possible that errors or omissions may occur in the content. The author and publishers assume no responsibility for, and give no guarantees or warranties concerning, the accuracy, completeness, or up-to-date nature of the information provided in this book.

CHAPTER 2

History Taking in General Practice

General Points

- In ideal circumstances, a psychiatric history is taken in quiet, unhurried surroundings. In practice, this rarely occurs, but it is still important to **optimise circumstances** as far as possible, with as few interruptions as feasible.
- Active listening is important: **paying genuine attention to someone for 10 minutes** is better than speaking distractedly with them for an hour.
- Be aware of your own **safety** and that of other staff and patients, especially if your patient is agitated or disturbed.

Presenting Complaint

- **What** has brought this person to see you? Common examples include 'low mood', 'feeling anxious', 'tired all the time', or 'my mother told me to come'.
- Are there any **relevant negatives**? For example, a patient who is depressed might not be suicidal.

Psychiatry Algorithms for Primary Care, First Edition. Gautam Gulati, Walter Cullen, and Brendan Kelly.
© 2021 John Wiley & Sons Ltd. Published 2021 by John Wiley & Sons Ltd.

History of Presenting Complaint

- **How long** has this being going on?
- Did anything **trigger** it? Why *now*?
- Is it getting **better or worse**?
- Has the patient tried any treatments themselves?

Past Psychiatric History

- Has this **happened before**? If so, what helped then?
- Does the patient have any **history of mental illness,** substance misuse, psychological treatments, or psychiatric hospitalisation? Ask specifically about psychological therapy or counselling.
- Has the patient ever self-harmed or **attempted suicide**? Or considered it?

Past Medical and Surgical History

- Has the patient had any major **medical or surgical problems**?
- In particular, is there any history of **epilepsy or head injury**?

Medication

- Is the patient on any **medication, either prescribed or over the counter**?
- Ask specifically about **contraception** and **injections** (e.g. depot antipsychotic medication).
- Is the patient **allergic** to anything?

Family History

- Is there any family history of **mental illness**, psychiatric hospitalisation, self-harm, or suicide?

- If so, does the patient know what treatments helped their family members?
- Do any particular illnesses or conditions run in the patient's family?

Personal History

- Is the patient aware of any health problems at **birth** or in childhood?
- How was the patient's **childhood** and **education**?
- Is there any history of **abuse** of any sort?
- Has the patient been **working** inside or outside the home in recent years?

Social History

- Where does the patient **live**, and with whom?
- What does the patient enjoy doing in their spare time?
- What is the patient's source of **income**?
- What is the patient's **relationship** status and do they have **children**?
- How many **pregnancies** have they had?
- Does the patient use **alcohol, cigarettes, or illegal drugs**?

Forensic History

- Has the patient ever been charged with an offence, appeared in court, been **convicted** of an offence, or spent a night in a police cell?
- Is the patient **currently facing charges** or investigation? Have they an upcoming court date for any reason?

Premorbid Personality

- How would the patient **describe themselves** before they developed their current complaint?
- How does the patient think **other people would describe them**?

CHAPTER 3

The Rapid Mental State Examination

General Points

- The mental state examination lies at the heart of assessment in psychiatry.
- The mental state examination starts from the moment you first have contact with the person and continues until the end of the consultation.
- It is useful to structure the mental state examination with care to ensure that all relevant information is recorded **systematically**.

Appearance and General Behaviour

- Is the person well dressed, with good **self-care**?
- Do they establish good **eye contact** and **rapport**?
- Is the person visibly depressed, distressed, anxious, or perplexed?

Speech

- Is the **rate** of speech fast or slow?
- Is the **volume** of speech too high, too low, or very changeable?

Psychiatry Algorithms for Primary Care, First Edition. Gautam Gulati, Walter Cullen, and Brendan Kelly.
© 2021 John Wiley & Sons Ltd. Published 2021 by John Wiley & Sons Ltd.

- Does the **tone** of the person's speech show good modulation or is their speech monotonous?
- Is the person's speech **unusual** in any other way?

Mood

- How does the person **subjectively** describe their mood? It can be useful to ask the person to rate their mood out of 10, where zero means very depressed and 10 means very happy.
- How do you **objectively** assess the person's mood to be? Depressed? Euthymic (normal)? Elated?

Affect

- How does the person **react** in the conversation to you?
- Are they normally reactive (nodding, smiling, etc.) or are their reactions blunted, muted, labile, or inappropriate?

Thought

- What are the chief themes of the person's **thought content**? Are they ruminating anxiously, brooding depressively, or thinking expansive, elated thoughts?
- Does the person have **delusions**, which are fixed beliefs that are culturally inappropriate and persist despite evidence to the contrary? Or do they have **over-valued ideas**, which are thoughts that are intrinsically culturally appropriate but are held to a degree that is not? Or **obsessions**, which are recurring thoughts that the person recognises as their own but cannot stop thinking? Or **intrusive thoughts**, that occur from time to time and cause the patient distress?
- Does the person have unusual thought form, also known as **thought disorder**? Do their thoughts move too quickly or too slowly? Do their thoughts follow logically from each other or jump inexplicably from theme to theme? Or does the person report that their thoughts are not their own, or are being read or affected by other people or outside forces?

- Does the person have **thoughts of harming themselves or others**? If so, how immediate are these thoughts and is the patient distressed by them? Suggested question: 'Are there times when things get so difficult that you feel that you can't carry on, that you want to end your life, or that you want to kill yourself?' Ask this question clearly, directly, and with both sympathy and focus. You need an answer. If the question is asked directly and without hesitation, patients will feel greatly relieved and will generally tell the truth.

Perception

- It is important to identify **hallucinations** (perceptions arising in the mind without an external stimulus, often associated with psychosis) or **illusions** (misperceptions of real stimuli, often associated with tiredness, anxiety, or poor lighting).
- Disturbances of perception can occur in any of the five senses: **hearing** (e.g. auditory hallucinations such as 'hearing voices' in schizophrenia); **vision** (e.g. simple visual hallucinations such as flashes of light or complex ones such as seeing faces); **touch** (e.g. a feeling of insects crawling on the skin in alcohol withdrawal); **smell** (e.g. unpleasant olfactory hallucinations in depression); or **taste** (e.g. gustatory hallucinations of a taste of poison in paranoia).
- **Hypnagogic** hallucinations (while falling sleep) or **hypnopompic** hallucinations (while waking up) do not generally indicate psychosis but can prove troublesome.

Cognition

- You gain an overall impression of a patient's cognition in general conversation.
- It is useful to check the person's **orientation in time, place, and person**.
- If more detailed assessment is needed, the **Mini-Mental State Examination** (MMSE) and **Montreal Cognitive Assessment** (MoCA) are both available online.

Insight

- Does the person **believe they are ill?**
- If so, do they believe they have **a physical or a mental illness?**
- Do they believe that **treatment will help?**
- Are they **willing to accept treatment?**

Resources

Mini-Mental State Examination (MMSE): https://bit.ly/2R0qbry
Montreal Cognitive Assessment (MoCA): https://bit.ly/343OHNK

PART 2

Common Psychiatric Disorders

CHAPTER 4

Generalised Anxiety Disorder (GAD)

Suspected GAD
- A patient presenting with 'excessive and uncontrollable worry' with associated motor tension, restlessness, irritability, poor sleep, and somatic symptoms (tachycardia, sweating, hyperventilation).
- A patient seeking reassurance about somatic symptoms or a chronic physical health condition.
- Anxiety symptoms typically 'free-floating' and not confined to a particular situation.
- Often comorbid with major depression, panic disorder, or OCD.

Duration of GAD
- A diagnosis of generalised anxiety requires > 6 months of symptoms.

Evaluate for Symptoms
- Excessive worry
- Dread
- Uneasiness
- Restlessness
- Tiredness
- Irritability
- Muscle tension
- Poor concentration
- Poor sleep
- Shortness of breath
- Tachycardia
- Sweating
- Dizziness

Evaluate for Impairment
- Social
- Occupational/Educational
- Domestic

Psychiatry Algorithms for Primary Care, First Edition. Gautam Gulati, Walter Cullen, and Brendan Kelly.
© 2021 John Wiley & Sons Ltd. Published 2021 by John Wiley & Sons Ltd.

Initiate Treatment

- In all cases, baseline blood tests including full blood count, urea and electrolytes, liver function tests, and thyroid function tests; rule out hypothyroidism.
- **Mild:** Avoid antidepressants. Individual non-facilitated self-help, individual guided self-help, psychoeducation groups, and monitoring.
- **Moderate:** Psychological treatment (CBT) or drug treatment (SSRI).
- **Severe:** Consider combination of antidepressants and psychological treatment and referral to secondary care.

Refer to Secondary Care

- Complex, treatment-refractory GAD
- Very marked functional impairment
- High risk of self-harm

Medication choice (see appendix on Commonly Prescribed Drugs for dosage)

	Comments	Caution
1st line		
SSRI (ideally sertraline or fluoxetine)	Well tolerated	May initially exacerbate anxiety symptoms. Start at lower dose. Hyponatremia, GI Bleeds in the elderly
SNRI (duloxetine or venlafaxine)	May help anxiety	Monitor BP with venlafaxine, may initially exacerbate anxiety symptoms. Start at lower dose. Sedation
Pregabalin	Can be given in divided doses	Response may be noted within first week of treatment
2nd line		
Agomelatine	May assist sleep	Needs monitoring of liver functions
Beta blockers (propranolol)	Useful for somatic symptoms (e.g. tachycardia)	Weight gain
Quetiapine	Can be used as monotherapy	
In crises		
Benzodiazepines	Short-term use only (max 2–4 weeks)	Risk of dependence

Warn patients about emergence of suicidal ideation with antidepressants.

Non-pharmacological interventions	
General advice for all patients	A healthy diet (particularly Mediterranean) Regular exercise Education Sleep hygiene Schedule pleasurable activities Contact numbers for support in crisis
Psychological interventions for mild GAD	Counselling in primary care, guided self-help, bibliotherapy, e.g. *Manage Your Mind*, 3rd edn, by Gillian Butler, Nick Grey, and Tony Hope (Oxford University Press, 2018).
Psychological interventions for moderate or severe GAD	Referral to a psychologist to consider a focused intervention such as CBT. Those with severe GAD may need to improve to be able to engage in some modalities of psychological therapy.

Also see algorithms for	**Self-Harm and Suicide** **Depression** **Commonly Prescribed Drugs**
Recommended reading	**1.** Taylor DM, Barnes TFE, & Young A, *The Maudsley Prescribing Guidelines in Psychiatry*, 13th edn (Hoboken, NJ; Chichester, UK: Wiley, 2018). **2.** NICE Guideline [CG113]: Generalised anxiety disorder and panic disorder in adults: management (first published 2011, last updated July 2019) (https://bit.ly/31hZp0f). **3.** HSE and ICGP, *Guidelines for the Management of Depression and Anxiety in Primary Care* (Irish College of General Practitioners, 2006) (https://bit.ly/2Zamk0s). **4.** Slee A, Nazareth I, Bondaronek P et al. Pharmacological treatments for generalised anxiety disorder: a systematic review and network meta-analysis. *The Lancet* 393;10173 (2019), 768–777 (https://doi.org/10.1016/S0140-6736(18)31793-8).

Resources

Beck Anxiety Inventory: https://bit.ly/3bIFtt4

Butler G, Grey N, & Hope T, *Manage Your Mind: The Mental Fitness Guide*, 3rd edn (Oxford University Press, 2018): https://bit.ly/2R71LN8

Mind: www.mind.org.uk

NHS website: https://www.nhs.uk/conditions/generalised-anxiety-disorder

CHAPTER 5

Panic Disorder

Suspected Panic Disorder

- A panic attack is an espisode of acute, intense anxiety, apprehension, and fear.
- Panic disorder is usually characterised by multiple unexpected panic attacks with persistent concern of future attacks.
- Panic disorder may or may not be accompanied by agoraphobia or other avoidance symptoms.
- The disorder is often co-morbid with depression and substance misuse.

Duration

- Attacks are unexpected/unpredictable and may last up to 45 minutes.
- If panic attacks occur in the context of depression, then depression should be considered the primary diagnosis.

Evaluate for Symptoms

- Dyspnea
- Dizziness
- Choking sensations
- Tremors
- Sweating
- Loss of balance or a feeling of faintness
- Palpitations or accelerated heart rate
- Nausea or other form of abdominal distress
- Depersonalisation or derealisation
- Paresthesias
- Hot flashes or chills
- Chest discomfort
- Fear of dying
- Fear of not being in control of oneself

Evaluate for Impairment

- Social
- Occupational/Educational
- Domestic

Psychiatry Algorithms for Primary Care, First Edition. Gautam Gulati, Walter Cullen, and Brendan Kelly.
© 2021 John Wiley & Sons Ltd. Published 2021 by John Wiley & Sons Ltd.

Initiate Treatment

- In all cases, baseline blood tests including full blood count, urea and electrolytes, liver function tests, and thyroid function tests; rule out hypothyroidism.
- Screen for nicotine, alcohol, caffeine, and recreational drug use.
- **Mild:** Avoid antidepressants. Individual non-facilitated self-help, individual guided self-help, psychoeducation groups, and monitoring. Encourage exercise.
- **Moderate to Severe:** Psychological treatment (CBT) is first line. Consider drug treatment (SSRI) if patient has not benefitted from psychological intervention or declined psychological intervention.

Refer to Secondary Care

- Lack of benefit from any two interventions in primary care
- Marked functional impairment
- High risk of self-harm

Medication choice (see appendix on Commonly Prescribed Drugs for dosage)

	Caution
1st line SSRI (such as Sertraline)	May initially exacerbate symptoms. Start at lower dose. Caution around hyponatremia and GI Bleeds in the elderly
Venlafaxine XR	Commence at a low dose
2nd line Mirtazapine	Weight gain, sedation
Avoid benzodiazepines save for acute crises	

Non-pharmacological interventions

General advice for all patients	A healthy diet (particularly Mediterranean) Regular exercise Education about panic disorder Contact numbers for support in crisis

Psychological interventions for mild panic disorder	Guided or individual self-help, support groups, bibliotherapy e.g. *Manage Your Mind*, 3rd edn, by Gillian Butler, Nick Grey, and Tony Hope (Oxford University Press, 2018). Anxiety management, e.g. relaxation training.
Psychological interventions for moderate or severe panic disorder	Referral to a psychologist to consider a focused intervention such as CBT. Those with severe panic disorder may need to improve to be able to engage in some modalities of psychological therapy.

Also see algorithms for	**Generalised Anxiety Disorder** **Depression**
Recommended reading	**1.** Taylor DM, Barnes TFE, & Young AH, *The Maudsley Prescribing Guidelines in Psychiatry*, 13th edn (Hoboken, NJ; Chichester, UK: Wiley, 2018).
	2. NICE Clinical guideline [CG113]: Generalized anxiety disorder and panic disorder in adults: management (published 2011, last updated July 2019) (https://bit.ly/2nXdVNq).
	3. HSE and ICGP, *Guidelines for the Management of Depression and Anxiety in Primary Care* (Irish College of General Practitioners, 2006) (https://bit.ly/2Zamk0s).
	4. Pompoli A, Furukawa TA, Imai H et al. Psychological therapies for panic disorder with or without agoraphobia in adults: a network meta-analysis. Cochrane Database of Systematic Reviews 2016, 4:CD011004 (https://doi.org/10.1002/14651858.CD011004.pub2).

Resources

Butler G, Grey N, & Hope T, *Manage Your Mind: The Mental Fitness Guide*, 3rd edn (Oxford University Press, 2018): https://bit.ly/2R71LN8
Mind: www.mind.org.uk
NHS website: https://www.nhs.uk/conditions/panic-disorder

CHAPTER 6

Obsessive Compulsive Disorder (OCD)

Suspected OCD
- A patient presenting with persistent and recurrent irrational thoughts (obsessions), resulting in marked anxiety and repetitive excessive behaviours (compulsions) as a means to reduce anxiety associated with obsessional thoughts.
- Often comorbid with depression.

Duration of Symptoms
- The obsessions or compulsions need to be time-consuming or cause clinically significant distress or impairment in social, occupational, or other important areas of functioning.
- The symptoms occur in 2 consecutive weeks.

Evaluate for Symptoms

Obsessional thoughts:
- fear of contamination
- fear of harm
- preoccupation with symmetry
- sacrilegious thoughts
- aggressive throughts

Compulsive acts, mental acts, or rituals:
- hand washing
- ordering
- checking
- praying
- counting
- repeating words
- repeating gestures
- hoarding

Evaluate for Impairment
- Social
- Occupational/Educational
- Domestic
- Evaluate for comorbid depression

Psychiatry Algorithms for Primary Care, First Edition. Gautam Gulati, Walter Cullen, and Brendan Kelly.
© 2021 John Wiley & Sons Ltd. Published 2021 by John Wiley & Sons Ltd.

Initiate Treatment

- **Mild functional impairment:** Consider referral for brief individual CBT (including ERP – exposure and response prevention) using structured self-help materials, by telephone, or group CBT (including ERP). Patients with an inadequate response should be offered the option of an SSRI or more intensive CBT.
- **Moderate functional impairment:** Consider SSRI or more intensive CBT.
- **Severe functional impairment:** Consider combination of SSRI and CBT and referral to secondary care.

Refer to Secondary Care

- Not responding to adequate trial on SSRI or clomipramine for a period of 3 months on a therapeutic dose.
- Concomitant depressive features or acute suicidal crisis.
- Severe and disabling symptoms.
- If uncertain about the risks associated with intrusive sexual, aggressive, or death-related thoughts; these themes are common in OCD and are often misinterpreted as indicating risk.

Medication choice in primary care

	Comments	Caution
1ˢᵗ line SSRI (ideally fluoxetine, paroxetine, fluvoxamine, sertraline, citalopram)	Dose required is higher than for treatment of depression If first SSRI is poorly tolerated or there is an inadequate response, review dose after 4–6 weeks; treat for 12 months if effective. Onset of effect may take up to 12 weeks	Hyponatremia, GI Bleeds in the elderly. Monitor for emergence or worsening of suicidal ideation
2ⁿᵈ line Clomipramine		ECG and blood pressure measurement if history of cardiovascular disease. Toxic in overdose so limit prescription if risk of self-harm

Also see algorithms for	**Generalised Anxiety Disorder** **Depression**
Recommended reading	1. Taylor DM, Barnes TFE, & Young AH, *The Maudsley Prescribing Guidelines in Psychiatry*, 13th edn (Hoboken, NJ; Chichester, UK: Wiley, 2018). 2. NICE Clinical guideline [CG31]: OCD and BDD: treatment (2005) (https://bit.ly/2oJc2V4). 3. HSE and ICGP, *Guidelines for the Management of Depression and Anxiety in Primary Care* (Irish College of General Practitioners, 2006) (https://bit.ly/2Zamk0s). 4. Skapinakis P, Caldwell DM, Hollingworth W et al. Pharmacological and psychotherapeutic interventions for management of obsessive-compulsive disorder in adults: a systematic review and network meta-analysis. *Lancet Psychiatry* 3;8 (2016), 730–739 (https://doi.org/10.1016/S2215-0366(16)30069-4).

Resources

NHS website: https://www.nhs.uk/conditions/obsessive-compulsive-disorder-ocd
Yale-Brown Obsessive Compulsive Scale (Y-BOCS): https://bit.ly/2X5CkQ4

CHAPTER 7

Social Phobia

Suspected Social Phobia	• A patient presenting with intense, irrational fear of social or performance situations in which the individual believes that he or she will be negatively scrutinised by others. • The individual recognises this reaction as either excessive or unreasonable. • Often comorbid with autism, depression, other anxiety disorders, and substance misuse.
Duration of Social Phobia	• Social situations almost always cause fear or anxiety associated with clinically significant distress or avoidance. • A diagnosis of social anxiety requires > 6 months of symptoms.
Evaluate for Symptoms	• Fear and avoidance of social situations. • Fear of perceived outcome in social situations (e.g. looking anxious, blushing, sweating, trembling, or appearing boring). • Anxiety symptoms. • Poor self-esteem. • Safety-seeking behaviours. • Anticipatory and post-event processing.
Evaluate for Impairment	• Social • Occupational/Educational • Domestic

Psychiatry Algorithms for Primary Care, First Edition. Gautam Gulati, Walter Cullen, and Brendan Kelly.
© 2021 John Wiley & Sons Ltd. Published 2021 by John Wiley & Sons Ltd.

Initiate Treatment

- Baseline blood tests – rule out hypothyroidism.
- If the person has only experienced significant social anxiety since the start of a depressive episode, treat the depression.
- Refer to primary care psychology.
- **CBT is the treatment of choice:** Avoid antidepressants. Do not routinely offer benzodiazepines, antipsychotics, or mindfulness-based interventions. Individual CBT is recommended by NICE based on the Clark and Wells model / Rapee and Heimberg model that recommends 14–15 individual sessions over 4 months.
- If patient declines CBT and wishes to consider another psychological intervention, offer CBT-based supported self-help. Another alternative is short-term psychodynamic psychotherapy over 6–8 months.
- **Use medication only if CBT not effective or patient declines psychological treatment:** 12-week trial of SSRI in the first instance, and can be in conjuction with CBT.

Refer to Secondary Care

- Complex, treatment-resistance
- Marked functional impairment
- High risk of self-harm
- For access to specialist psychological services

Medication choice		
	Comments	**Caution**
1st line		
SSRI (escitalopram or sertraline) 10–12 week trial	Well tolerated	Hyponatremia, GI Bleeds in the elderly
SSRI (paroxetine or fluvoxamine)		Paroxetine can cause initial increase in agitation and also withdrawal effects on discontinuation. Fluvoxamine has hepatic liver-enzyme related drug interactions.
2nd line		
SNRI (venlafaxine modified release)		Monitor BP
3rd line		
MAOI (moclobemide, phenelzine)		Problematic interactions / strict diet

Warn patients about emergence of suicidal ideation with antidepressants

Also see algorithms for	**Self-Harm and Suicide** **Panic Disorder** **Depression**
Recommended reading	1. Taylor DM, Barnes TRE, & Young AH, *The Maudsley Prescribing Guidelines in Psychiatry*, 13th edn (Hoboken, NJ; Chichester, UK: Wiley, 2018). 2. NICE Clinical guideline [CG159]: Social anxiety disorder: recognition, assessment and treatment (2013) (https://bit.ly/2r2SifV). 3. HSE and ICGP, *Guidelines for the Management of Depression and Anxiety in Primary Care* (Irish College of General Practitioners, 2006) (https://bit.ly/2Zamk0s). 4. American Psychiatric Association, *Diagnostic and Statistical Manual of Mental Disorders*, 5th edn (DSM-5) (Arlington, VA: APA Publishing, 2013). 5. Stein MB, & Stein DJ. Social anxiety disorder. *The Lancet* 371:9618 (2018), 1115–1125 (https://doi.org/10.1016/S0140-6736(08)60488-2).

Resources

CCI (Australia) self-help resource for patients: https://bit.ly/2X9fxCN
NHS website: https://www.nhs.uk/conditions/social-anxiety

CHAPTER 8

Post-Traumatic Stress Disorder (PTSD)

Suspected PTSD
- A patient presenting with episodes of repeated reliving of a traumatic episode through intrusive memories or 'flashbacks', nightmares, avoidance of activities associated with trauma, and autonomic hyperarousal.
- Arises as a delayed or protracted response to a single or multiple threatening or catastrophic event.

Duration
- There is usually a latency period of a few weeks to months between trauma and onset of symptoms.
- A diagnosis of PTSD requires > 1 month of symptoms.

Evaluate for Symptoms
- Re-experiencing or 'flashbacks'
- Nightmares
- Dissociation
- Anhedonia
- Emotional blunting
- Poor concentration
- Avoidance of situations reminiscent of experienced trauma
- Hyperarousal (including hypervigilance, anger, and irritability)
- Enhanced startle reaction

Evaluate for Impairment
- Social
- Occupational/Educational
- Domestic
- Evaluate for comorbid depression

Psychiatry Algorithms for Primary Care, First Edition. Gautam Gulati, Walter Cullen, and Brendan Kelly.
© 2021 John Wiley & Sons Ltd. Published 2021 by John Wiley & Sons Ltd.

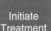

Initiate Treatment

Primary treatent modality is psychological – consider referral to a psychologist for:
- Individual trauma-focused CBT to adults who have presented more than 1 month after traumatic event.
- EMDR (eye movement desensitisation reprocessing) for adults 1–3 months after recent trauma, if the patient has a preference for this.
- EMDR for adults with a diagnosis of PTSD or symptoms of PTSD > 3 months after recent trauma.

Medication:
- Consider SSRI (sertraline) or SNRI (venlafaxine) for patients with PTSD who express a preference for drug treatment.
- Consider antipsychotics (such as risperidone) in addition to psychological therapies if experiencing disabling symptoms and behaviours, or psychosis.

Refer to Secondary Care

- Complex, treatment-refractory PTSD
- Very marked functional impairment
- High risk of self-harm

Antidepressant choice		
	Comments	**Caution**
1st line SSRI (paroxetine, sertraline, or fluoxetine) Venlafaxine XR	Well tolerated	Hyponatremia, GI Bleeds in the elderly Monitor BP with venlafaxine. May initially exacerbate anxiety symptoms. Start at lower dose
2nd line Amitriptyline Mirtazapine Antipsychotics (risperidone, olanzapine, quetiapine)	May assist sleep Effective for intrusive symptoms (flashbacks, nightmares)	Toxic in overdose Weight gain, sedation Weight gain, sedation

Also see algorithms for	**Depression**
Recommended reading	1. Taylor DM, Barnes TRE, & Young AH, *The Maudsley Prescribing Guidelines in Psychiatry*, 13th edn (Hoboken, NJ; Chichester, UK: Wiley, 2018).
	2. NICE Guideline [NG116]: Post-traumatic stress disorder overview (2018) (https://bit.ly/3eamp82).
	3. HSE and ICGP, *Guidelines for the Management of Depression and Anxiety in Primary Care* (Irish College of General Practitioners, 2006) (https://bit.ly/2Zamk0s).
	4. Karatzias, T, Murphy, P, Cloitre, M et al. Psychological interventions for ICD-11 complex PTSD symptoms: systematic review and meta-analysis. *Psychological Medicine* 49;11 (2019), 1761–1775 (https://doi.org/10.1017/S0033291719000436).

Resources

Combat Stress – veterans' mental health (UK): www.combatstress.org.uk

MIND – self-care for PTSD: https://bit.ly/2xO4DHT

NHS website: https://www.nhs.uk/conditions/post-traumatic-stress-disorder-ptsd

CHAPTER 9

Depression

Suspected Depression
- A patient presenting as 'down, depressed, or hopeless' or with a 'lack of interest or enjoyment'.
- Higher index of suspicion if they, or a family member have had depression in the past, if the patient has significant social stressors, a serious physical illness, misuses drugs or alcohol, or is postpartum.

Duration of Symptoms
- A diagnosis of depression requires > 2 weeks of symptoms.
- If less than 2 weeks, consider an adjustment reaction, provide support and monitor.

Evaluate for Symptoms
- Low mood
- Loss of interest/enjoyment
- Lack of energy
- Reduced appetite
- Reduced sleep
- Reduced sex drive
- Reduced concentration
- Thoughts of self-harm or suicide
- Hopelessness
- Feelings of guilt
- Somatic symptoms without an underlying cause
- Psychotic symptoms such as nihilistic delusions, auditory hallucinations
- Any history of elated mood? (beware of bipolar disorder)

Evaluate for Impairment
- Social
- Occupational/Educational
- Domestic

Psychiatry Algorithms for Primary Care, First Edition. Gautam Gulati, Walter Cullen, and Brendan Kelly.
© 2021 John Wiley & Sons Ltd. Published 2021 by John Wiley & Sons Ltd.

Establish Diagnosis and Severity

- **Mild:** 1–2 symptoms and some difficulty in continuing with activities.
- **Moderate:** 4–5 symptoms and considerable difficulty in continuing with activities.
- **Severe:** Several symptoms or the presence of psychosis or significant suicidal ideation; unlikely to be continuing with activities or to a very limited extent.

Initiate Treatment

- In all cases, baseline blood tests including full blood count, urea and electrolytes, liver function tests and thyroid function tests; rule out hypothyroidism.
- Review medication list for source of iatrogenic depression, e.g. beta blockers.
- **Mild:** Avoid antidepressants. Psychoeducation, support, advice on diet and exercise. Consider referral for counselling.
- **Moderate:** Consider antidepressant or psychological treatment or combination.
- **Severe:** Consider combination of antidepressants and psychological treatment and referral to secondary care.

Refer to Secondary Care

- Moderate depression not responding to two trials of antidepressants at adequate dosage.
- Severe depression with psychotic symptoms or acute suicidal crisis.
- Treatment resistant depression.
- Suspected bipolar affective disorder.

Antidepressant choice (see appendix on Commonly Prescribed Drugs for dosage)

	Comments	Caution
1st line		
Ideally SSRI e.g. sertraline or escitalopram	Well tolerated	Hyponatremia, GI Bleeds in the elderly
Or NaSSa such as mirtazapine	May assist sleep	Weight gain
Or SNRI such as duloxetine or venlafaxine	May help anxiety	Monitor BP with venlafaxine

2nd line		
Try alternative from 1st line choices before		SSRIs have the best tolerability
Tricyclic such as amitriptyline		Toxic in overdose
MAOI such as tranylcypromine		Problematic interactions/strict diet
3rd line		
Vortioxetine/ agomelatine		Agomelatine requires liver function monitoring
Augmentation e.g. lithium or antipsychotic or combination antidepressants	Best done in consultation with secondary care	

Treatment timeframes	
After adequate therapeutic dose of an antidepressant, if not effective, switch to another after assessing for	2 weeks
After switching antidepressant and titrating to a therapeutic dose, assess over	3–4 weeks
After recovery from a single episode, continue treatment for	6–9 months
After recovery from a second or further episode, particularly with significant impairment, continue treatment for at least	2 years

Warn patients about emergence of suicidal ideation with antidepressants.

Non-pharmacological interventions	
General advice for all patients	A healthy diet (particularly Mediterranean)
	Regular exercise
	Education about depression
	Sleep hygiene
	Schedule pleasurable activities
	Contact numbers for support in crisis

Psychological interventions for mild depression	Counselling in primary care, guided self-help, bibliotherapy e.g. *Manage Your Mind*, 3rd edn, by Gillian Butler, Nick Grey, and Tony Hope (Oxford University Press, 2018)
Psychological interventions for moderate or severe depression	Referral to a psychologist to consider a focused intervention such as CBT or interpersonal therapy Those with severe depression may need to improve to be able to engage in some modalities of psychological therapy

Also see algorithms for	**Self-Harm and Suicide** **Generalised Anxiety Disorder** **Bipolar Affective Disorder** **Commonly Prescribed Drugs**
Recommended reading	1. Taylor DM, Barnes TFE, & Young AH, *The Maudsley Prescribing Guidelines in Psychiatry*, 13th edn (Hoboken, NJ; Chichester, UK: Wiley, 2018). 2. NICE Clinical guideline [CG90]: Depression in adults: recognition and management (2009) (https://bit.ly/1sS6Uuo). 3. HSE and ICGP, *Guidelines for the Management of Depression and Anxiety in Primary Care* (Irish College of General Practitioners, 2006) (https://bit.ly/2Zamk0s). 4. Malhi GS, & Mann JJ. Depression. *The Lancet* 392;10161 (2018), 2299–2312 (https://doi.org/10.1016/S0140-6736(18)31948-2).

Resources

Beck's Depression Inventory: https://bit.ly/2ynCack
Butler G, Grey N, & Hope T, *Manage Your Mind: The Mental Fitness Guide*, 3rd edn, (Oxford University Press, 2018): https://bit.ly/2R71LN8
Mind: www.mind.org.uk
NHS website: http://www.nhs.uk/conditions/depression

CHAPTER 10

Bipolar Affective Disorder (BPAD)

Suspected BPAD

- An ICD-10 diagnosis of bipolar disorder requires at least two episodes in which mood and activity levels are significantly disturbed, being, on some occasions, an elevation of mood with increased energy and activity (i.e. hypomania or mania, also known as 'elation') and on other occasions a lowering of mood with decreased energy and activity (depression).
- Lesser changes in mood might be normal mood variations; 'cyclothymia', in which mood fluctuations are greater than normal but insufficient for a diagnosis of bipolar disorder; or bipolar II, with milder mood elevations alternating with depression.

Evaluate for Symptoms

Mania in bipolar disorder:
- *Hypomania* involves persistent mild elevation of mood, increased activity, enhanced energy, marked talkativeness, over-familiarity, and excessive feelings of well-being.
- *Mania without psychotic symptoms* is characterized by elation, overactivity, pressure of speech, reduced need for sleep, inflated self-esteem, and disinhibition.
- *Mania with psychotic symptoms* involves a significant break with reality in at least one respect, often involving grandiose delusions or mood-congruent hallucinations.

Depression in bipolar disorder:
- Characteristic symptoms include depressed mood, loss of enjoyment, diminished interest, reduced energy, decreased activity and increased fatiguability.
- There may also be thoughts or acts of self-harm and suicidality.
- Depression in bipolar disorder can be indistinguishable from recurrent depressive disorder, so careful history-taking for past episodes of mania is vital.

Evaluate for Impairment

- Social
- Occupational/Educational
- Domestic

Psychiatry Algorithms for Primary Care, First Edition. Gautam Gulati, Walter Cullen, and Brendan Kelly.
© 2021 John Wiley & Sons Ltd. Published 2021 by John Wiley & Sons Ltd.

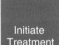

Investigations in suspected bipolar disorder:
- Full history, asking especially for previous episodes of mania or depression.
- Collateral history, from family or friends.
- Mental state examination, with particular emphasis on mood, suicidality, features of psychosis, and insight.
- Drug testing, if indicated (e.g. for cocaine, cannabis, steroids).
- Physical investigations, if a physical cause is suspected (e.g. thyroid disease).

Treatment of mania in bipolar disorder:
- If the person is taking a mood-stabilising medication such as lithium, check adherence, plasma level, and any other medication that might be affecting it.
- If the person is taking an antidepressant on its own, consider stopping it and offer an antipsychotic medication such as haloperidol, olanzapine, quetiapine, or risperidone.
- If the person is not taking an antipsychotic or mood-stabiliser, offer an antipsychotic.
- Further steps in treatment, if needed, will likely require specialist mental health services input (e.g. further alternative antipsychotics or adding a mood-stabiliser).
- When prescribing, take account of the person's preferences, advance statements, and relevant clinical factors (e.g. previous response, side effects, physical comorbidity).

Treatment of depression in bipolar disorder:
- Psychological therapy for depression is very helpful in bipolar disorder, especially in terms of avoiding triggering a manic episode.
- If a person develops moderate or severe bipolar depression and is not taking medication for bipolar disorder, offer fluoxetine (antidepressant) with olanzapine, or else quetiapine on its own. (If the person is already on lithium, optimise lithium first)
- Further steps in treatment will likely require specialist mental health services input.

Initiate Treatment

Refer to Secondary Care
- Specialist secondary care is usually required, at least initially, for bipolar disorder, but ongoing management is often provided in primary care.
- Psychotic symptoms are usually sufficient reason for referral; additional reasons include disturbed behavior, suicidality, treatment resistance, or failure of outpatient care.

Maintenance treatment in bipolar disorder:
- Lithium is the first-line, long-term treatment for bipolar disorder; if it is ineffective, valproate can be added (but not in women of child-bearing age).
- If lithium is poorly tolerated or unsuitable, valproate or olanzapine can be used, or else quetiapine (if it has been effective for an episode of mania or bipolar depression).
- If these approaches do not produce sufficient improvement, specialist treatments are required (e.g. combinations of medications, electroconvulsive therapy), especially for rapid-cycling (four or more mood episodes within a year).

Maintenance treatment with lithium:

- Maintain plasma lithium levels between 0.6 and 0.8 mmol per litre for people on lithium for the first time; and between 0.8 and 1.0 for those previously on lithium.

- Measure plasma lithium level weekly initially and following dose changes, until the level stabilises; then every 3 months for a year; and then every 6 months.

- Continue 3-monthly monitoring in older adults; people taking drugs that interact with lithium; people at risk of impaired renal or thyroid function, raised calcium levels, or other complications; people with poor symptom control or poor adherence; and people whose last lithium level was 0.8 mmol per litre or greater.

- Measure weight, kidney function, calcium, estimated glomerular filtration rate and thyroid function at least every 6 months.

- Monitor for side-effects: hand tremor; increased thirst and urination; diarrhoea and vomiting; weight gain; impaired concentration and memory; drowsiness; muscle weakness; acne; hair loss; and hypothyroidism.

- Monitor for lithium toxicity (a medical emergency): side-effects (see above), slurred speech, heightened reflexes, tachycardia, hyperthermia, agitation, seizures, kidney failure, uncontrollable eye movements, hypotension, confusion, coma, delirium, death.

QTc prolongation resulting from antipsychotic medication:

- The QTc interval reflects the duration of cardiac repolarization, corrected for heart rate.

- QTc is prolonged if it exceeds 440 milliseconds in men or 470 milliseconds in women.

- QTc of greater than 500 milliseconds is associated with increased risk of **torsades de pointes** and cardiac death.

- QTc should be recorded when starting an antipsychotic and annually thereafter.

Ongoing treatment of bipolar disorder:

- Psychoeducation enhances the therapeutic alliance.

- Psychological approaches assist many patients and families to manage the disorder.

- Physical healthcare is vital: stopping smoking, improved diet and lifestyle, and screening for cardiac risk-factors (e.g. cholesterol, high blood pressure).

Also see algorithms for	**Self-Harm and Suicide** **Generalised Anxiety Disorder** **Depression**
Recommended reading	1. Taylor DM, Barnes TFE, & Young AH, *The Maudsley Prescribing Guidelines in Psychiatry*, 13th edn (Hoboken, NJ; Chichester, UK: Wiley, 2018). 2. NICE Clinical guideline [CG185]: Bipolar disorder: assessment and management (2018) (https://bit.ly/3bLgG7H).

Resources

Mind: www.mind.org.uk

NHS website: http://www.nhs.uk/conditions/bipolar-disorder

Price P, *The Cyclothymia Workbook: Learn How to Manage Your Mood Swings and Lead a Balanced Life* (Oakland, CA: New Harbinger Publications, Inc., 2004): https://bit.ly/2UHljtS

CHAPTER 11

Psychosis

Suspected Psychosis

- 'Positive' symptoms include delusions (fixed, false, culturally inappropriate beliefs that persist despite contrary evidence), hallucinations (perceptions without external stimuli), and thought disorder (unusual thought form, block or interference).
- Negative symptoms include difficulties concentrating, anxiety, depressed mood, poor sleep, suspiciousness, and social withdrawal.
- Presentations vary greatly, ranging from quiet, paranoid delusions persisting for years to sudden-onset commanding auditory hallucinations.

Duration of Symptoms

- Psychosis can be caused by schizophrenia, schizoaffective disorder, severe depression, severe mania (in bipolar disorder), delusional disorder, alcohol or substance misuse (when not intoxicated or withdrawing), organic disorders (e.g. brain tumours), trauma, stress, or the side-effects of medication.
- An ICD-10 diagnosis of schizophrenia requires either one major symptom or two minor symptoms to be present for most of the time during an episode of psychotic illness lasting for at least one month, or else at some time during most of the days.

Evaluate for Symptoms

- Thought echo (hearing one's thoughts spoken aloud), believing thoughts are inserted or withdrawn from one's head or are broadcast.
- Delusions that one's thoughts, actions, feelings, or perceptions are controlled by someone or something else.
- Hearing voices give a running commentary on your behaviour, having discussions about you among themselves, or emanating from your body.
- Other persistent delusions that are culturally inappropriate and impossible (e.g. having superhuman powers).
- Persistent hallucinations of any sort, every day for some weeks, accompanied by delusions (which may be fleeting) without apparent explanation.
- Difficulties with clear thinking, such as sudden interruptions of thoughts, resulting in diminished coherence.
- Changes in muscle tone, such as stiffness or apparent inability to operate one's muscles and/or limbs in the normal fashion, possibly resulting in complete lack of movement ('catatonia').
- 'Negative symptoms' such as reduced speech, emotions, energy or interest, or social withdrawal.

Psychiatry Algorithms for Primary Care, First Edition. Gautam Gulati, Walter Cullen, and Brendan Kelly.
© 2021 John Wiley & Sons Ltd. Published 2021 by John Wiley & Sons Ltd.

Evaluate for Impairment

- Social
- Occupational/Educational
- Domestic

Management

Management of psychosis:
- *Investigations:* Collateral history (all cases), brain imaging (if an organic cause, such as tumour or head injury, is suspected).
- *Treatment will depend on cause:* Depressive psychosis may require antipsychotic and/or antidepressant medication; severe mania in bipolar disorder may require antipsychotic and/or mood-stabilising medication; schizophrenia will likely require antipsychotic medication and a range of other measures; and substance use may require antipsychotic medication in the short term and rehabilitation in the longer term.

Treatment of schizophrenia:
- Early intervention is recommended with antipsychotic medication in conjunction with psychological interventions (e.g. family interventions, CBT).
- 6-week trial of an 'atypical' antipsychotic medication.
- If this does not produce satisfactory clinical results, assess adherence.
- If adherence is satisfactory, try a 6-week trial of another atypical or a typical antipsychotic (tablets or injections)
- If this does not produce sufficient clinical improvement, specialist treatments in secondary care are required (e.g. combinations, clozapine, electroconvulsive therapy).

Refer to Secondary Care

- Psychotic symptoms alone are usually sufficient reason for referral, but additional reasons include disturbed behavior, suicidality, treatment resistance, or failure of outpatient care.
- Specialist secondary care is usually required for specific groups such as children with psychosis, people with co-morbid intellectual disability, patients with paraphrenia (organised delusional systems without deterioration of intellect or personality), and post-partum mental illness (which can involve psychosis).

Antipsychotic choice

Medication choice	Comments	Caution
'Atypical' or 'second generation' antipsychotic medications: e.g. risperidone, olanzapine, quetiapine, aripiprazole, amisulpride, ziprasidone, paliperidone	Side effects can include weight gain, impaired glucose tolerance, diabetes mellitus, dry mouth, sedation, possible cardiac effects, dizziness, impotence	Prior to any antipsychotic, every patient should have an ECG, weight and height check, and basic blood tests, including blood glucose. Monitor these annually
'Typical' or 'first generation' antipsychotic medications: e.g. fluphenazine, flupentixol, haloperidol, zuclopenthixol, sulpiride, pimozide	Side effects can include movement problems (e.g. restlessness); metabolic, cardiac, or hormonal effects (e.g. raised prolactin)	With all antipsychotics, 'neuroleptic malignant syndrome' can occur; this is a rare adverse effect (pyrexia, confusion, muscle rigidity, perspiration, tachycardia) that needs hospital management and can be fatal

QTc prolongation resulting from antipsychotic medication:

- The QTc interval reflects the duration of cardiac repolarization, corrected for heart rate.
- QTc is prolonged if it exceeds 440 milliseconds in men or 470 milliseconds in women.
- QTc of greater than 500 milliseconds is associated with increased risk of torsades de pointes and cardiac death.

Ongoing treatment of schizophrenia:

- There is a high risk of relapse if medication is stopped within one to two years.
- Psychoeducation enhances the therapeutic alliance.
- Psychological approaches of proven benefit include CBT, family therapy, art therapy, social support, occupational therapy, and self-help groups.
- Physical healthcare is vital: stopping smoking, improved diet and lifestyle, and screening for cardiac risk-factors (e.g. cholesterol, high blood pressure).

Also see algorithms for	**Substance Misuse**
Recommended reading	1. Taylor DM, Barnes TFE, & Young AH, *The Maudsley Prescribing Guidelines in Psychiatry*, 13th edn (Hoboken, NJ; Chichester, UK: Wiley, 2018). 2. NICE Clinical guideline [CG178]: Psychosis and schizophrenia in adults: prevention and management (2014) (https://bit.ly/2wepjsi). 3. NICE Technology appraisal guidance [TA59]: Guidance on the use of electroconvulsive therapy (2009) (https://bit.ly/39KfSyH).

Resources

Hearing Voices Network: www.hearing-voices.org
Mind: www.mind.org.uk
NHS website: http://www.nhs.uk/conditions/psychosis

CHAPTER 12

Eating Disorders

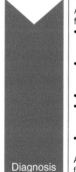

Diagnosis

An ICD-10 diagnosis of **anorexia nervosa** requires all five of the following criteria:
- Body weight maintained at least 15% below expected body weight or a body-mass index (BMI) of 17.5 or less (BMI is weight in kilograms divided by height in metres squared, i.e. kg/m^2).
- Weight loss is self-induced by avoiding foods seen as 'fattening'; there may also be self-induced vomiting or purging, excessive exercise, and use of appetite suppressants or diuretics.
- Body-image distortion with a dread of 'fatness'.
- Endocrine dysfunction such as amenorrhoea, loss of sexual interest and potency, and disorders of growth hormone, cortisol, thyroid hormone, and insulin secretion.
- If onset is pubertal, pubertal events are delayed or arrested.

An ICD-10 diagnosis of **bulimia nervosa** requires all three of the following criteria:
- Persistent preoccupation with eating and an insatiable craving for food.
- Efforts to counteract the 'fattening' effect of food by self-induced vomiting, abuse of purgatives, periods of starvation, appetite suppressants, and other methods.
- Morbid dread of 'fatness' and setting a target weight well below a healthy weight.

Other eating disorders include atypical anorexia nervosa, atypical bulimia nervosa, binge eating disorder, obesity, orthorexia (an obsession with proper or 'healthful' eating), over-eating in association with other psychological disturbances (e.g. bereavements) and vomiting in association with other psychological disturbances (e.g. dissociation or hypochondriasis).

Psychiatry Algorithms for Primary Care, First Edition. Gautam Gulati, Walter Cullen, and Brendan Kelly.
© 2021 John Wiley & Sons Ltd. Published 2021 by John Wiley & Sons Ltd.

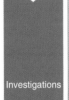

Investigations

- *Full history*, asking especially for previous symptoms relating to eating and early problems with food.
- *Collateral history*, from family, friends or others, as indicated.
- *Physical examination*, with particular emphasis on height, weight, heart rate, blood pressure, temperature, skin, nails, and cardiovascular examination; distinctive signs of anorexia nervosa include emaciation, dry skin, fine lanugo hair (on trunk and face), hypotension, bradycardia, and evidence of repeated vomiting (pitted teeth, parotid swelling, and scarring on the dorsum of the hand, known as Russell's sign).
- *Mental state examination*, with particular emphasis on mood, suicidality, attitudes towards food, insight, and willingness to engage in treatment.
- *Physical investigations*, including full blood count, renal function, liver function, thyroid function, urinalysis and other tests as indicated (e.g. ECG, X-rays to examine bones); common laboratory abnormalities include anaemia, leucopenia, hypokalemia, and alkalosis.
- *Drug testing*, if indicated, for illegal drugs, appetite suppressants, diuretics, or steroids.

Refer to Secondary Care

- Specialist secondary care is usually required, at least initially, for eating disorders, although much ongoing management and monitoring is often provided in primary care, including management of family anxieties.
- Additional reasons for referral to secondary medical or psychiatric care include severe weight loss, widespread endocrine disturbance, electrolyte imbalance, disturbed behaviour, suicidality, treatment resistance, or failure of outpatient care.

Physical healthcare in eating disorders:

- *Electrolyte abnormalities* such as hypokalemia require immediate attention as they may be life-threatening.

- In general terms, *weight restoration* should be steady rather than dramatic in order to avoid 're-feeding' problems (e.g. hypophosphataemia) and to maintain the therapeutic alliance.

- *Specialist mental health services input* is usually required and inpatient care may be indicated if weight loss is rapid and severe, BMI is less than 13.5 (owing to high risk of fatal arrhythmia and hypoglycaemia), there is significant risk of suicide or there are physical sequelae of purging or starvation.

Psychological treatment of eating disorders:

- *Eating-disorder-focused cognitive behavioural therapy* (CBT-ED) is recommended as the mainstay of treatment for anorexia nervosa and is accessed through specialist mental health services.

- CBT-ED usually comprises up to 40 therapy sessions over 40 weeks, with twice-weekly sessions in the first 2 or 3 weeks, with the aim of reducing the risk to physical health and addressing other symptoms of the eating disorder.

- CBT-ED is also used for bulimia nervosa and binge eating disorder if guided self-help is unacceptable, contraindicated or ineffective after four weeks.

- Other models of psychotherapeutic care can also be used, especially for children, and these are generally provided by specialist mental health services.

Pharmacological treatment:

- *Antidepressants* (e.g. fluoxetine 60 mg daily) are sometimes used for bulimia nervosa and binge eating disorder, but appear less effective than psychological therapy, are not a substitute for psychological therapy, and are usually prescribed by specialist services.

Also see algorithms for	**Self-Harm and Suicide** **Generalised Anxiety Disorder** **Depression**
Recommended reading	1. NICE Guideline [NG69]: Eating disorders: recognition and treatment (2017) (https://bit.ly/2UzYV5C). 2. Taylor DM, Barnes TRE, & Young AH, *The Maudsley Prescribing Guidelines in Psychiatry*, 13th edn (Hoboken, NJ; and Chichester: Wiley, 2018).

Resources

Beat Eating Disorders: www.beateatingdisorders.org.uk
Mind: www.mind.org.uk
NHS website: http://www.nhs.uk/conditions/eating-disorders

CHAPTER 13

Personality Disorders

Presentations
- Acute stress, inappropriate demands, disproportionate anger, frequent conflicts
- Recurring symptoms of mood or anxiety disorder
- Self-harm
- Problem substance abuse
- Medically unexplained symptoms

Duration
- To make a diagnosis, clinical features should have been evident developmentally by early adulthood and should be persistent, trait-like. They should be evident in a variety of situations, over time. They should be associated with significant social, domestic, or occupational impairment.

Evaluate for Symptoms

See 'Diagnostic Considerations' – some symptoms include:
- Paranoia
- Odd thinking
- Restricted range of emotions
- Anger and irritability
- Excessive emotionality
- Anxiety
- Impulsive behaviour
- Grandiosity
- Self-harm

Assessment
- Risk factors include: (i) history of abuse, (ii) family history of schizophrenia/negative parenting interactions, (iii) disruptive disorder as a child.
- People do not present seeking relief from personality difficulties.
- Symptoms relate to cognitive-perceptual problems, affective dysregulation, impulse control, and can result in difficulties in interpersonal interactions.
- While all encounters viewed as 'difficult' are not confirmation of a personality disorder, repeated such encounters may suggest the diagnosis be considered.

Psychiatry Algorithms for Primary Care, First Edition. Gautam Gulati, Walter Cullen, and Brendan Kelly.
© 2021 John Wiley & Sons Ltd. Published 2021 by John Wiley & Sons Ltd.

Initiate Treatment

- Acutely, may need to explore suicidality and assess risk.
- Aim to establish a stable, supportive relationship with patient.
- Psychotherapy and other psychosocial interventions can help patients with relationship issues, to confront fears, cope with trauma, deal with dysfunctional thoughts, e.g. CBT, mindfulness, dynamic psychotherapy, dialectical behaviour therapy, mentalisation-based therapy, transference-focused psychotherapy. Some of these may be available in primary care but often require specialist referral.
- Psychotropic medication treatment is not generally recommended. However, depression and anxiety when co-morbid is treated with SSRI antidepressants. Off licence low dose antipsychotic treatment with olanzapine (2.5–5 mg) or quetiapine (25–50 mg) is sometimes used as a short-term prescription to help emotional regulation in crises although a safer alternative would be low dose promethazine (25–50 mg). Quasi-psychotic symptoms may sometimes require treatment with low dose antipsychotics.
- Patient communication and relationship management strategies.
- Substance abuse, particularly alcohol abuse, is often co-morbid and requires treatment.

Refer to Secondary Care

- Mangement of self-harm risk.
- For access to specialist psychological treatment such as dialectical behaviour therapy (DBT).
- For detailed assessment of personality disorder traits and approach to medical care in complex presentations.

Diagnostic considerations:

- Pervasive patterns of maladaptive behaviour, cognition, and inner experience.
- Deviating from cultural norms and associated with significant distress or disability.
- Begin by early adulthood and present in many contexts.
- Occur in 9–11% of general population.

Eleven types of personality disorder which can be grouped into three broad clusters:

Cluster	Personality disorder	DSM-5 definition
A	Schizotypal	Social and interpersonal deficits marked by acute discomfort with / reduced capacity for close relationships; cognitive or perceptual distortions and eccentricities of behaviour
	Schizoid	Detached from social relationships, restricted range of emotions
	Paranoid	Distrust and suspiciousness of others such that their motives are interpreted as malevolent

B	Borderline	Pervasive pattern of instability in interpersonal relationships, self-image and affect, markedly impulsive behavior, efforts to avoid abandonment, chronic feelings of emptiness, recurrent self-harm, suicidal gestures or threats
	Histrionic	Excessive emotionality and attention-seeking
	Antisocial	Disregard for others beginning at age 15, impulsivity, deceitfulness; lack of remorse, engages in acts that are illegal, disrespect for social norms
	Narcissistic	Grandiosity, need for admiration, lack of empathy, views self as 'special' and needs to be admired
C	Avoidant	Widespread pattern of inhibition around people, feeling inadequate and sensitive to negative evaluation
	Dependent	Need to be taken care of leading to submissive and clinging behaviour and fears of separation
	Obsessive compulsive	Preoccupation with perfectionism, orderliness, interpersonal/mental control, at the cost of efficiency, flexibility, and openness
Not otherwise specified		Disorder of personality functioning that does not meet criteria for any specific personality disorder; may have features of more than one personality disorder

Note: General practitioners may benefit from discussing with peer groups and within 'Balint' groups (see Resources). Practitioner self-care is often relevant in managing these disorders.

Also see algorithms for	**Self-Harm and Suicide** **Generalised Anxiety Disorder** **Depression**
Recommended reading	1. American Psychiatric Association, *Diagnostic and Statistical Manual of Mental Disorders*, 5th ed. (DSM-5) (Washington, DC: APA Publishing, 2013). 2. Angstman KB, & Rasmussen NH. Personality disorders: review and clinical application in daily practice. *Am Fam Physician.* 2011 Dec 1;84(11):1253–1260. Review. 3. NICE Quality standard [QS88]: Personality disorders: borderline and antisocial (2015) (https://bit.ly/3emKQ1U). 4. Schrift MJ, Personality disorders. *BMJ Best practice* (last updated January 2019) (https://bit.ly/3eghK4h).

Resources

NHS website: https://www.nhs.uk/conditions/borderline-personality-disorder

Salinksy J, *A very short introduction to Balint groups* (The Balint Society, 2009): https://bit.ly/3bFLpDc

Ward RK, Assessment and management of personality disorders. *Am Fam Physician.* 2004 Oct 15;70(8):1505–1512: https://bit.ly/3bosdKx

CHAPTER 14

Alcohol Use Disorder

Suspected Alcohol Use Disorder

- Consider Alcohol Use Disorder in all patients.
- Especially consider screening new patients, patients with relevant physical (liver or cardiac disease) or mental (depression, anxiety) illnesses, during antenatal appointments, patients who have been assaulted, those seeking help with their alcohol use.

Assessment and Stratification

- Use AUDIT-C as a screen (https://bit.ly/2LP9kpG), if score <= 4 indicates drinking at safe level if > 5 perform full AUDIT (also at https://bit.ly/2LP9kpG).
- AUDIT will sort patients into lower risk (0–7), increasing risk (8–15), higher risk (16–19), and possible dependence (>= 20).

Management

- Lower risk – reinforce benefits of lower-risk drinking.
- Increasing risk – offer a brief intervention and advice in respect of cutting down.
- Higher risk – referral for counselling, advice on Alcoholics Anonymous / 12-step programmes.
- Possible dependence – further assessment and referral to specialist services as a dependence syndrome is possible.

Additional Considerations

- Quantify alcohol use over previous 30 days and ask about other drugs / substances.
- Consider using Severity of Alcohol Dependence Questionnaire SADQ-C (https://bit.ly/2OorkJ6): a score over 16 usually indicates that chlordiazepoxide detoxification may need to be considered. The usual regimen is 20 mg QDS reduced over 5–7 days. Higher doses may be needed in more severe cases.
- Assess for signs of physical or mental illnesses (see Depression, Anxiety), MMSE if cognitive decline suspected.
- Consider FBC (raised MCV), LFTs (raised GGT), prothrombin time, viral screen.
- Prescribe thiamine in cases of harmful use and dependence: 200–300 mg daily in divided doses during assisted withdrawal or in patients drinking excessively.
- Assess readiness for change.

Psychiatry Algorithms for Primary Care, First Edition. Gautam Gulati, Walter Cullen, and Brendan Kelly.
© 2021 John Wiley & Sons Ltd. Published 2021 by John Wiley & Sons Ltd.

Refer to Secondary Care

- To a general hospital / specialist residential centre for detoxification with intravenous thiamine and oral benzodiazepines, particularly in those with a history of seizures or delirium tremens, physical comorbidities, malnutrition, cognitive decline, or comorbid learning disability.
- To a medical specialist if there is liver dysfunction or pancreatitis.
- To psychiatric services where there is comorbid moderate or severe depression evident 3–4 weeks after abstinence.
- For residential rehabilitation for support with maintaining abstinence after detoxification in cases of dependence particularly where there is homelessness and support is needed to find accommodation.

Medication for relapse prevention and/or reduction of alcohol consumption (all are specialist initiated or advised)

	Comments	Caution
Acamprosate	Anticraving drug 666mg tds (bd if < 60kg) for 6–12 months	Pregnancy / breast feeding, severe kidney disease, severe liver disease
Naltrexone	Anticraving and relapse prevention Start after detox 25mg daily increasing to maintenance 50mg daily for 6–12 months	Stop if drinking persists 4–6 weeks after starting
Disulfiram	Start > 24 hours after last alcoholic drink Dose 200mg daily	Provokes unpleasant (and potentially severe) reaction if alcohol consumed concomitantly Can cause flushing, nausea, palpitations, arrhythmias, hypotension, and collapse
Nalmefene	18mg once daily with monthly review for ongoing benefit and a maximum treatment duration of 1 year	Contraindicated in severe renal or severe hepatic impairment

Non-pharmacological interventions	
Brief intervention	Opportunistic – delivered in empathetic and non-judgemental way
	Advice covering potential harm and the benefits of reducing/stopping, barriers to change
	Practical suggestions on how to reduce alcohol consumption including community support networks and AA
	Leads to a set of goals
	With or without formal follow up
	Up to 10 minutes in duration
FRAMES: Brief advice in primary care	**Feedback:** provide feedback on the patient's risk for alcohol problems
	Responsibility: highlight that the individual is responsible for change
	Advice: advise reduction or give explicit direction to change
	Menu: provide a variety of options for change
	Empathy: emphasise a warm, reflective, and understanding approach
	Self-efficacy: encourage optimism about changing behaviour

Also see algorithms for	**Depression**
	Generalised Anxiety Disorder
	Substance Use Disorder
Recommended reading	1. Taylor DM, Barnes TFE, & Young AH, *The Maudsley Prescribing Guidelines in Psychiatry*, 13th edn (Hoboken, NJ; Chichester, UK: Wiley, 2018).
	2. NICE Clinical guideline [CG115]: Alcohol use disorders (2011) (https://bit.ly/1I76q5r).
	3. Anderson P, O'Donnell A, & Kaner E. Managing alcohol use disorder in primary health care. *Curr Psychiatry Rep.* 2017 Sep 14;19(11):79 (https://doi.org/10.1007/s11920-017-0837-z).

Resources

AUDIT-C Questions and AUDIT (Alcohol Use Disorders Identification Test):
  https://bit.ly/2LP9kpG
Severity of Alcohol Dependence Questionnaire SADQ-C: https://bit.ly/2OorkJ6

CHAPTER 15

Substance Use Disorder

Suspected Substance Use Disorder
- Consider Substance Use Disorder screening in new patients, patients with relevant physical (liver, cardiac, or infectious disease) or mental (depression, anxiety) illnesses, during antenatal appointments, and in patients belonging to marginalised groups (homeless, former prisoners, migrants, and refugees).

Assessment and Stratification
- Use DUDIT as a screen (https://bit.ly/366uO8K), consider CUDIT-R (https://bit.ly/2PhqjBz) for specific cannabis screening.
- DUDIT will sort male patients into low risk (0–5), harmful use (6–25), or likely dependence (> 25).
- Female patients who score > 1 will require assessment for harmful use.

Management
- Low risk – reinforce benefits of lower drug consumption.
- Harmful use – offer a brief intervention and advice in respect of cutting down, refer to local drug treatment service for support.
- Dependence – complete a comprehensive assessment with a view to making a referral to secondary care.

Additional Considerations
- Quantify substance use over previous 30 days including alcohol use.
- Assess for signs of physical illness, including withdrawal symptoms.
- Consider urine drug screen, pregnancy test, hepatitis, and HIV virology.
- Assess for signs of comorbid mental illnes, depression, anxiety, and psychosis.
- Assess readiness for change and motivation to engage with addiction services.

Referral
- Patients who are using drugs but do not meet the criteria for dependence may still benefit from referral to addiction services or a voluntary sector support service for advice and support.
- Patients meeting criteria for dependence may benefit from residential treatment especially if previous community stabilisation has not been effective or their circumstances are chaotic.
- Patients meeting criteria for dependence and consenting to referral should be referred to the appropriate healthcare service or voluntary sector service.

Psychiatry Algorithms for Primary Care, First Edition. Gautam Gulati, Walter Cullen, and Brendan Kelly.
© 2021 John Wiley & Sons Ltd. Published 2021 by John Wiley & Sons Ltd.

Drug misuse	
	Specific considerations
Amphetamine	There is no evidence that substitution therapy helps. Treatment of withdrawal is symptomatic. Drug-induced psychosis may need treatment with antipsychotics
Benzodiazepine	Patients who misuse or have been on long-term benzodiazepine prescriptions may experience a withdrawal syndrome if abruptly discontinued. Prevention is important – these medications should ideally only be prescribed for short trials of 2–3 weeks
	When tapering prescriptions of benzodiazepines, consider switching to a drug with a longer half-life such as diazepam and reduce the dosage by an eighth every fortnight aiming to cease the drug within 6 months
Cannabis	There is no evidence that substitution therapy helps. Treatment of withdrawal is symptomatic. Drug-induced psychosis may need treatment with antipsychotics
Cocaine	There is no evidence that substitution therapy helps. Treatment of withdrawal is symptomatic. Drug-induced psychosis may need treatment with antipsychotics
GHB (γ-hydroxybutyrate)	Withdrawal syndrome can be severe – may mimic alcohol withdrawal but progress to severe physical complications, psychosis, and delirium. Consider inpatient treatment – seek specialist care. Diazepam and muscle relaxants may be helpful
Opiate	See specific algorithm. Opiate substitution treatment, e.g. with methadone and buprenorphine, is a specialist area

Also see algorithms for	**Alcohol Use Disorder** **Opiate Use Disorder** **Depression** **Generalised Anxiety Disorder**
Recommended reading	1. Health Service Executive, *Clinical Guidelines for Opioid Substitution Treatment* (Dublin: HSE, 2017) (https://bit.ly/2RrnFvu). 2. O'Shea, J, Goff, P, & Armstrong, R, *SAOR: Screening and Brief Intervention for Problem Alcohol and Substance Use*, 2nd edn (Dublin: Health Service Executive, 2017) (https://bit.ly/2PnpWFB). 3. A list of local services for treatment in Ireland can be found at www.drugs.ie. 4. Taylor DM, Barnes TFE, & Young AH, *The Maudsley Prescribing Guidelines in Psychiatry*, 13th edn (Hoboken, NJ; Chichester, UK: Wiley, 2018). 5. NICE Quality standard [QS23]: Drug use disorders in adults (2011) (https://bit.ly/2LJ9dvx). 6. Department of Health & Social Care, *Drug Misuse and Dependence: UK Guidelines for Clinical Management* (London: DHSC, 2017) (https://bit.ly/33Wp1Ru).

Resources

Cannabis Use Disorder Identification Test – CUDIT-R: https://bit.ly/2PhqjBz
Drug Use Disorder Identification Test DUDIT: https://bit.ly/366uO8K
RCGP substance misuse toolkit: https://bit.ly/2Rdcxl9

CHAPTER 16

Opiate Use Disorder

Opioid substitution treatment (OST)	
Dependence	• To commence OST (methadone or buprenorphine), a patient must meet ICD-10 criteria for dependence (e.g. withdrawal, tolerance, difficulty controlling use, continued use despite harms, time spent seeking opioids or recovering from the same, neglect of important social, occupational, or recreational activities) • Obtain a urine sample and test for opioids, including specific heroin metabolite 6-AM if appropriate. Consider urine pregnancy test
Signs of withdrawal	• Consider using the Clinical Opiate Withdrawal Scale (https://bit.ly/34Uzm1K) • Physical signs – yawning, coughing, sneezing, runny nose, lachrymation, raised blood pressure, increased pulse, dilated pupils, cool, clammy skin, diarrhoea, nausea, fine muscle tremor • Psychological – restlessness, agitation, anxiety, sleep disturbance, dysphoria, craving
General health assessment	• Comprehensive history, check for previous drug and alcohol use and treatments, identify current polydrug use • Drug-related physical problems, e.g. abscesses, venous thrombosis, septicemia • Hepatitis A, B, and C virology and evidence of immunizations where appropriate, sexually transmitted infections, ECG if cardiac risk factors for QT prolongation risk

Psychiatry Algorithms for Primary Care, First Edition. Gautam Gulati, Walter Cullen, and Brendan Kelly.
© 2021 John Wiley & Sons Ltd. Published 2021 by John Wiley & Sons Ltd.

Referral (will vary by jurisdiction)	• If clinically indicated the patient can be referred to a specialist GP or a specialist addiction clinic • The Central Treatment List (CTL, Ireland) will verify the patient is not already registered for OST • The patient will be then placed on the national waiting list until an appropriate place is available • Priority is given to pregnant women, under-18s, patients with HIV and serious illnesses, and those who have detoxified and recently relapsed • The CTL will issue a treatment card allowing the patient to receive OST at a named pharmacy
Follow up	• The patient will attend the nominated addiction service or specialist GP for their OST and OST specific care (e.g. virology) • This service should liaise with referring GP on other health matters • The subsequent phases of OST are induction, stabilisation, maintenance, and detoxification • Stable patients in the maintenance phase can be referred back to the referring GP

This is a specialist area. There is a risk of opioid overdose during the induction of opioid substitution if the starting dosage is too high, or if there is concomitant misuse of opioids or other central nervous system depressants.

An opioid overdose can be recognised by pinpoint pupils, respiratory rate < 8, unconsciousness, cyanosis, cold skin. This is an emergency. In addition to CPR and calling 999, administration of naloxone 400mcg IM should be considered.

Also see algorithms for	**Substance Use Disorder**
Recommended reading	1. Health Service Executive, *Clinical Guidelines for Opioid Substitution Treatment* (Dublin: HSE, 2017) (https://bit.ly/2RrnFvu). 2. Taylor DM, Barnes TFE, & Young AH, *The Maudsley Prescribing Guidelines in Psychiatry*, 13th edn (Hoboken, NJ: Chichester, UK: Wiley, 2018). 3. NICE Quality standard [QS23]: Drug use disorders in adults (2012) (https://bit.ly/2LJ9dvx). 4. Department of Health & Social Care, *Drug Misuse and Dependence: UK Guidelines for Clinical Management* (London: DHSC, 2017) (https://bit.ly/33Wp1Ru).

Resources

Clinical Opiate Withdrawal Scale: https://bit.ly/34Uzm1K
RCGP Guidance on the use of substitute prescribing in the treatment of opioid dependence in primary care: https://bit.ly/2UYDMB0

CHAPTER 17

Adult Attention Deficit Hyperactivity Disorder (ADHD)

Suspected ADHD
- A patient presenting a history of childhood treatment for ADHD or with symptoms that indicate pervasive problems with inattention, impulsivity, and hyperactivity / 'mental restlessness'.
- Higher index of suspicion if a family member has a diagnosis of ADHD and in those wih a history of preterm birth, neurodevelopmental conditions, conduct disorder or epilepsy.

Duration of Symptoms
- Did symptoms begin in childhood and appear to persist throughout adulthood?

Screen for Symptoms
- Use a standardised self-rating scale such as the Adult ADHD Self-Report Scale (accessible at https://bit.ly/1PM6kpG). If there are four or more darkly shaded boxes in Part A, suspect a diagnosis of ADHD.
- If in doubt about the childhood onset of symptoms, use a scale that measures childhood recall of symptoms such as the Wender Utah Rating Scale (accessible at https://bit.ly/39IcqEN). Use a cut-off of 46.
- Exclude alternative psychiatric illness that could explain the presentation.

Evaluate for Impairment
- Social, Domestic, or Occupational/Educational disruption particularly in two or more areas.

Psychiatry Algorithms for Primary Care, First Edition. Gautam Gulati, Walter Cullen, and Brendan Kelly.
© 2021 John Wiley & Sons Ltd. Published 2021 by John Wiley & Sons Ltd.

Refer to Secondary Care
- All adults with suspected ADHD should be referred to secondary care for diagnosis and management.
- Include in the referral letter any history of tics or seizures or any cardiac history as well as any history of substance misuse.
- Diagnosis should be established only by a specialist, who may use validated instruments such as the DIVA-5 (Diagnostic Interview for ADHD in Adults: https://bit.ly/2wJWsJn).

Initiating Treatment
- Treatment initiation is in secondary care but often requires the general practitioner to carry out a physical examination including baseline weight, height, blood pressure, pulse, cardiac auscultation, ECG, full blood count, urea and electrolytes and liver function tests.
- Medication is advised by secondary care with requests for monitoring the above parameters.
- Patients once established on effective medication and connected to additional resources are often discharged to primary care for ongoing prescription.

Request Annual Review by Secondary Care
- If stable, re-refer to secondary care on an annual basis.
- All patients on ADHD medication should be reviewed in secondary care on an annual basis to see if they still meet criteria for diagnosis and for medication review.

Medication (always initiated in secondary care)		
	Comments	**Caution**
1st line (6-week trial of either)		
Dexamfetamine or lisdexamfetamine	Short acting so can be easily titrated	Avoid where there is a risk of diversion. Monitor for aggression, tics
Methylphenidate	Available in short-, medium-, and long-acting preparations	Avoid where there is a risk of diversion. Monitor for depression, appetite changes, tics
2nd line Atomoxetine	Safer where diversion is a risk and used first line in this scenario	Avoid if significant cardiac disease. Monitor for suicidal ideation. Baseline ECG needed. Monitor liver function tests
3rd line Guanfacine, modafinil	Tertiary care	

Non-pharmacological interventions	
General advice for all patients	A healthy balanced diet
	Regular exercise
	Education about Adult ADHD
	Sleep hygiene
	Support with substance misuse if this is a comorbidity
	Contact for support organisations, such as the ADHD Foundation which has advice on self-help (https://bit.ly/2XmrEtL)
Occupational interventions	This is usually done in secondary care through involvement of an occupational therapist to evaluate and advise on education and employment
Psychological interventions	This is usually done in secondary care through involvement of a psychologist for group-based CBT

Also see algorithms for	Special Considerations: Children and Adolescents
Recommended reading	**1.** Taylor DM, Barnes TFE, & Young AH, *The Maudsley Prescribing Guidelines in Psychiatry,* 13th edn (Hoboken, NJ; Chichester, UK: Wiley, 2018).
	2. NICE Guideline [NG87]: ADHD: diagnosis and management (2019) (https://bit.ly/2TMU6nr).
	3. Kooij SJJ, Bejerot S, & Blackwell A et al. European consensus statement on diagnosis and treatment of adult ADHD: The European Network Adult ADHD. *BMC Psychiatry* 10;67 (2010) (https://doi.org/10.1186/1471-244X-10-67).

Resources

ADHD Foundation: https://bit.ly/2XmrEtL
Adult ADHD Self Report Scale ASRS-v1.1: https://bit.ly/1PM6kpG
Wender Utah Rating Scale for ADHD: https://bit.ly/39IcqEN

CHAPTER 18

Autism Spectrum Disorder (ASD)

When to Suspect ASD
- ASD may be suspected where there are persistent difficulties in social interaction, social communication, and a restricted repertoire of interests and activities accompanied by difficulties in education/occupation or relationships.
- Sensory difficulties with noise/light/touch are often an initial indicator of the disorder.
- It is frequently comorbid with intellectual disabilities or neurodevelopmental conditions.

Screening
- A useful screening tool is the Autism Spectrum Quotient AQ-10 – a 10-item scale (https://bit.ly/2NDa82g). Use a cut-off of 6.
- For individuals with moderate to severe intellectual disability ascertain whether there is evidence of the following: limited interaction: lack of responsiveness in social situations; little or no change in behaviour in different social situations; rigid routines; resistance to change; repetitive activities such as rocking, hand or finger flapping (particularly when stressed).

Refer to Secondary Care
- Refer to a specialist in secondary care experienced in ASD to establish diagnosis and necessary supports.
- This is specialist area and ASD-specific teams or specialists in intellectual disabilities may be involved in assessments.
- Family and/or carer involvement is beneficial.

Prescribing for Core Symptoms
- There is no role for antipsychotics, antidepressants, anticonvulsants, or exclusion diets in respect of core symptoms of ASD.
- Melatonin has some evidence for ASD-related sleep disturbance.

Psychiatry Algorithms for Primary Care, First Edition. Gautam Gulati, Walter Cullen, and Brendan Kelly.
© 2021 John Wiley & Sons Ltd. Published 2021 by John Wiley & Sons Ltd.

Prescribing for Challenging Behaviour

- Avoid using medication as first line for challenging behaviour.
- Exclude physical causes such as pain, reflux, or constipation.
- Assess for possible mental illness.
- Involve specialist teams to evaluate and modify the environment, to perform functional analysis of behaviour, and to determine a psychosocial treatment plan.
- Low-dose antipsychotics (risperidone, aripiprazole) when used should be commenced by specialists.

Monitoring of Medication

- Where antipsychotics are used in challenging behaviour, their efficacy must be reevaluated within 3–4 weeks with discontinuation in 6 weeks if there is no benefit.
- In addition, patients with ASD on antipsychotics should be monitored for somnolence, metabolic syndrome, hyperprolactinemia, and for reductions in seizure threshold when there is comorbid epilepsy.

Also see algorithms for	**Generalised Anxiety Disorder** **Special Considerations: People with Intellectual Disabilities**
Recommended reading	1. Bhaumik S, Gangadharan SK, Braford D, & Barrett M, *The Frith Prescribing Guidelines for People with Intellectual Disability*, 3rd edn (Chichester, Uk: Wiley, 2015). 2. NICE Clinical guideline [CG142]: Autism spectrum disorder in adults: diagnosis and management (2016) (https://bit.ly/32aHyZT). 3. Matson et al. Issues in the management of challenging behaviour in adults with an autism spectrum disorder. *CNS Drugs* 25 (2011), 597–606 (https://doi.org/10.2165/11591700-000000000-00000).

Resources

AQ-10 screening test: https://bit.ly/2xvIVZB
RCGP Autistic Spectrum Disorders Toolkit: https://bit.ly/34EHGDJ

CHAPTER 19

Delirium

Risk Factors
- Delirium is an acute change in cognitive function that has an organic cause and is likely to be reversible.
- Risk factors include cognitive impairment (past or present) and/or dementia, age > 65 years, multiple physical comorbidities particularly neurological or cerebrovascular, pharmacological treatment of psychiatric comorbidities, history of delirium, polypharmacy, recent hospitalisation.

Making the Diagnosis
- Acute onset over 24–48 hours and a fluctuating course.
- Disturbance of consciousness (reduced awareness of the environment).
- A change in cognition (reduced concentration, poor responses, memory deficit, disorientation, language disturbance) not better explained by a pre-existing/progressing dementia.
- Disturbance of perception (auditory or visual hallucinations).
- Changes in physical function (reduced mobility, reduced movement, restlessness, agitation, changes in appetite, sleep disturbance).
- Changes in social behaviour (lack of cooperation to reasonable requests, withdrawal).

- If indications of delirium (above) are identified, a standardised clinical assessment tool such as the Confusion Assessment Method (CAM) (https://bit.ly/3frGMia) can be used to confirm the diagnosis.

Investigations
- Seek to find and treat the underlying cause(s). A physical and neurological examination may be supplemented by excluding constipation and urinary retention. Look for evidence of pain or infection. Assess hydration level. Review medication lists for recent changes. Any recent discharge from hospital, recent discontinuation of alcohol or sedative, or change in environment?
- Blood tests may include a full blood count, liver profile, renal profile, electrolytes, calcium, magnesium, phosphate and inflammatory markers, blood glucose, and thyroid function tests.

Psychiatry Algorithms for Primary Care, First Edition. Gautam Gulati, Walter Cullen, and Brendan Kelly.
© 2021 John Wiley & Sons Ltd. Published 2021 by John Wiley & Sons Ltd.

Management
- Non-pharmacological strategies should be instituted. These include consistent nursing, preventing sensory deprivation, reorientation, familiar environments.
- Pharmacological treatment should be directed primarily at the underlying cause and then at the relief of specific symptoms of delirium.
- For agitation and/or distress, use verbal or non-verbal de-escalation. If these fail, low-dose haloperidol may be considered.

Refer to Secondary Care
- If the primary cause of delirium requires general hospital care. Remember – untreated delirium carries high mortality.
- If delirium persists and a source of the cause for the delirium cannot be identified.
- If delirium does not resolve despite non-pharmacological measures or despite pharmacological treatment of underlying cause.

Pharmacological treatment		
Antipsychotics (note increased risk of stroke in patients with dementia)		
Drug	**Oral dose**	**Adverse effects**
1ˢᵗ line Haloperidol	0.5–1mg BD	Monitor for extra pyramidal side effects and prolonged QT interval
Olanzapine	2.5–5mg per day (do not exceed 20mg in 24 hours)	Monitor for sedation
Risperidone	Oral 0.5mg BD (do not exceed 4mg in 24 hours)	Monitor for hypotension and extrapyramidal side effects
1ˢᵗ line Quetiapine	Oral 12.5–50mg BD (do not exceed 200mg in 24 hours)	Monitor for sedation and postural hypotension

Benzodiazepines (note association with prolongation/ worsening of symptoms)		
Lorazepam (Avoid except for use in alcohol/sedative withdrawal, Lewy Body Dementia, Parkinson's disease and Neuroleptic Malignant Syndrome)	Oral 0.25–1mg every 2–4 hours as needed (do not exceed 3mg in 24 hours)	Monitor for respiratory depression, over-sedation, and paradoxical excitement

Also see algorithms for	**Dementia**
Recommended reading	1. Taylor DM, Barnes TFE, & Young AH, *The Maudsley Prescribing Guidelines in Psychiatry,* 13th edn (Hoboken, NJ; Chichester, UK: Wiley, 2018).
	2. NICE Clinical guidelines [CG103]: Delirium: prevention, diagnosis and management (first published 2010, last updated 2019) (https://bit.ly/2HuljYI).
	3. Royal Australian College of General Practitioners, *Medical Care of Older Persons in Residential Aged Care Facilities,* 4th edn (Melbourne, Australia: RACGP, 2006).
	4. British Geriatrics Society, CGA in primary care settings: patients presenting with confusion and delirium (2019) (https://bit.ly/2kw1Hd1).

Resources

Confusion Assessment Method (CAM): https://bit.ly/2lQ57Y0
HSE Early Identification and Initial Management of Delirium in the Emergency Department (includes 4AT screening instrument): https://bit.ly/3aCeEH1

CHAPTER 20

Dementia

Suspected Dementia

- Progressive, largely irreversible clinical syndrome with global deterioration in cognitive function, behaviour, and personality (with normal consciousness, perception).
- Most common types: Alzheimer's disease, vascular dementia, mixed dementia, dementia with Lewy bodies, and frontotemporal dementia.
- Often the presenting complaint is one of 'forgetfulness'.

Evaluate for Symptoms

History:
- Age, family history.
- Progression of condition, associated myoclonus, seizures, depression, anxiety.
- Medical/psychiatric history, e.g. diabetes, hypertension, CVA.
- Toxin exposure, e.g. alcohol, lead, drugs.
- Risk factors – age, learning disability, female gender, family history, alcohol consumption, smoking, obesity, head injury, hypertension, hyperlipidemia.

Cognition and functional impairment:
- Decline in recent memory, repetitive questioning, difficult to recall date/time.
- Difficulty performing complex tasks, judgement, planning, analytic thought, finding one's way around familiar places (spatial awareness), language impairment (problems expressing themselves / getting lost in conversations).
- Challenging behaviour, symptoms such as depression, agitation, disinhibition, psychosis, wandering, aggression, incontinence.
- Basic tasks of self-care.

Examination:
- Mental state examination – to identify depression or non-cognitive symptoms due to dementia.
- Cognitive examination, standardised screening tests include.
  - 30-item Mini Mental State Examination (MMSE)
  - General Practitioner Assessment of Cognition (GPCOG)
  - Montreal Cognitive Assessment (MoCA)
  - Mini-Cog
- Physical examination to exclude other causes (focal neurological deficits, stepwise course, skin/hair changes, postural instability).

Psychiatry Algorithms for Primary Care, First Edition. Gautam Gulati, Walter Cullen, and Brendan Kelly.
© 2021 John Wiley & Sons Ltd. Published 2021 by John Wiley & Sons Ltd.

| **Evaluate for Impairment** | • Functional impairment – 'Informant Questionnaire on Cognitive Decline in the Elderly (IQCODE)' when taking collateral history. |

| **Investigations** | • FBC, ESR, CRP,T4, TSH, Biochemistry – liver, renal, bone, glucose, B12, folate.
• Midstream urine test and chest X Ray if delirium is a possibility.
• Consider electrocardiogram (ECG necessary if starting acetylcholinesterase inhibitor).
• Other tests (not routine in primary care) include: syphilis, HIV, caeruloplasmin.
Other **specialist** investigations include:
• Imaging to exclude other cerebral pathologies (e.g. subdural haematoma, normal pressure hydrocephalus, cerebral tumours) and to establish dementia subtype.
• Single-photon emission computed tomography (SPECT) to differentiate Alzheimer's disease, vascular dementia, and frontotemporal dementia.
• More rarely, EEG, CSF, brain biopsy. |

| **Refer to Secondary Care** | • If reversible causes of cognitive decline have been investigated.
• Dementia is rapidly progressive.
• For imaging, especially if atypical presentation, rapid deterioration, unexplained focal neurological signs, head injury, urinary incontinence, gait ataxia. |

Treatment

Non-pharmacological:

- Information and advice about the disease, treatments, support services, financial/legal advice, driving.
- Cognitive stimulation, i.e. engage in activities that involve cognitive processing, such as 'structured group cognitive stimulation therapy'.
- Reality orientation therapy (if disoriented in time, place, and person).

Pharmacological therapy for Alzheimer's disease:

- Acetylcholinesterase inhibitors (donepezil, galantamine, and rivastigmine) for mild/moderate disease.
- Memantine for more severe disease (or if other medicines not tolerated).

Drug treatments for behavioural problems in dementia (seek specialist advice):

- Mild agitation: trazodone, lorazepam, citalopram, sertraline.
- Severe agitation or psychosis: quetiapine, risperidone, olanzapine, aripiprazole.
- Depressive symptoms: citalopram, sertraline, mirtazapine.

The use of psychotropics in the elderly requires particular caution, e.g. QT prolongation on ECG, increased risk of GI Bleeds with some SSRIs, increased risk of cerebrovascular events with some atypical antipsychotics. The risk of falls and postural hypotension is a particular risk. Consider non-pharmacological strategies, be aware of risks of polypharmacy and underlying medical conditions, refer to an up-to-date formulary and seek specialist advice.

Also see algorithms for	Delirium **Special Considerations: The Elderly** **Commonly Prescribed Drugs**
Recommended reading	1. Neugroschl J, Alzheimer's dementia. *BMJ Best Practice* (last updated 2 May 2019) (https://bit.ly/39Etqvl). 2. Burns A, & Iliffe S. Dementia. *BMJ* 2009;338:b75 (https://doi.org/10.1136/bmj.b75). 3. NICE Guideline [NG97]: Dementia: assessment, management and support for people living with dementia and their carers (2018) (https://bit.ly/2xKHp5A).

Resources

30-item Mini Mental State Examination (MMSE): https://bit.ly/3dTexbN
General Practitioner Assessment of Cognition (GPCOG): https://bit.ly/2V4oBGG
Informant Questionnaire on Cognitive Decline in the Elderly (IQCODE): https://bit.ly/2BPAef3
Mini-Cog: https://bit.ly/2V0TXh1
Montreal Cognitive Assessment (MOCA): https://bit.ly/3bRPS5T

PART 3

Common Presentations in Primary Care

CHAPTER 21

Fatigue

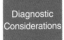

Diagnostic Considerations
- Sensation of exhaustion during/after usual activities, or feeling of inadequate energy to begin activities.
- 4–13% in general population; 11–33% in general practice.
- Six most common causes are (in order): viral illness, upper respiratory infection, iron-deficiency anaemia, acute bronchitis, medication effects, depression (psychological).
- Step-wise approach to assessment is important.

Characterise the Fatigue
- Duration (recent, prolonged, or chronic).
- Sudden/progressive.
- Impact of physical or mental activity.
- Level of physical activity (sedentary lifestyle is a cause of fatigue, and patients may benefit from exercise therapy).
- Concomitant muscle weakness (e.g. suggests neuromuscular disorder).
- Seasonality (may suggest viral).

Check for Underlying Disease
- Age over 60 years.
- Recent sore throat (EBV infection) or fever / cough / sore throat (influenza infection).
- Menorrhagia (anaemia).
- Polyuria, polydipsia (diabetes).
- Cold intolerance, overweight (hypothyroid) or heat intolerance, weight loss (hyperthyroid).
- Weight loss, blood in stool (malignancy, anaemia).
- Exposure to infections (e.g. TB, brucellosis, toxoplasmosis, Lyme disease) due to work, travel, or contact with animals.
- Immunosuppression.
- Intravenous drug use or unprotected sexual intercourse (HIV / hepatitis infection).
- Cardiovascular / respiratory risk factors / symptoms.
- Steatorrhoea / weight loss (coeliac disease).
- Arthralgia or rash (autoimmune disease).
- Neurological symptoms.
- Medicines, e.g. antiarrhythmics, antidepressants, anti-emetics, anti-epileptics, antihistamines, antihypertensives, corticosteroids, diuretics, neuroleptic agents.

Psychiatry Algorithms for Primary Care, First Edition. Gautam Gulati, Walter Cullen, and Brendan Kelly.
© 2021 John Wiley & Sons Ltd. Published 2021 by John Wiley & Sons Ltd.

Check for Psychiatric Disorders
- Most commonly depression, but also anxiety disorders, somatisation disorders.
- Alcohol / substance use disorders.
- Insomnia / sleep problems.

Refer to Secondary Care
- For investigations as necessary.
- If 'red flags' – weight loss, lymphadenopathy, symptoms of malignancy (e.g. haemoptysis, dysphagia, rectal bleeding, breast lump, postmenopausal bleeding), focal neurological signs, sleep apnoea, features of inflammatory arthritis / connective tissue disease / cardiorespiratory disease.

Physical examination:

- General appearance (psychomotor impairment, poor grooming).
- Lymphadenopathy.
- Pallor, tachycardia, blueish sclera, systolic ejection murmur suggest anaemia.
- Then, examination as suggested by other symptoms, e.g. cardiorespiratory examination (COPD, asthma, heart failure), neurological examination (especially tone, power).

Investigations:

- Initial tests include FBC (and differential), ESR, CRP, biochemistry (renal, liver, calcium, phosphate), fasting blood glucose, TSH, urinalysis.
- Subsequent tests (if indicated) may include: Monospot, ECG, cardiac enzymes, CXR, toxicology, cortisol, HIV/hepatitis serology, tuberculin test, ANA, TTG/EMA, anti-mitochondrial antibodies, BNP, serum heavy metals.
- Investigations for underlying malignancy may include: CXR, imaging (abdomen/pelvis), cytology/biopsy. Abnormal FBC (film/differential) may indicate bone marrow aspiration.

Fatigue syndromes:

- Chronic fatigue syndrome: Fatigue lasting >6 months plus four of the following: memory impairment, tender lymph nodes, myalgia, arthralgia, headache, unrefreshing sleep, post-exertional malaise (>24 h).
- Chronic fatigue: Clinically evaluated unexplained chronic fatigue with no obvious medical cause that fails to meet the criteria for chronic fatigue syndrome.

Also see algorithms for	**Insomnia** **Substance Use Disorder** **Alcohol Use Disorder** **Depression**
Recommended reading	1. Favrat B, Cornuz J. Assessment of fatigue. *BMJ Best practice* (last updated May 2020) (https://bit.ly/2JNeuR3). 2. Cornuz J, Guessous I, & Favrat B. Fatigue: a practical approach to diagnosis in primary care. *CMAJ.* 2006 Mar 14;174(6):765–767 (https://doi.org/10.1503/cmaj.1031153). 3. Hamilton W, Watson J, & Round A. Investigating fatigue in primary care. *BMJ.* 2010 Aug 24;341:c4259 (https://doi.org/10.1136/bmj.c4259). 4. NICE Clinical guideline [CG53]: Chronic fatigue syndrome/myalgic encephalomyelitis (or encephalopathy); diagnosis and management (2007) (https://bit.ly/2yGxFtI).

Resources

Alcohol Use Disorders Identification Test (AUDIT): https://bit.ly/2UMRRmg
Patient Health Questionnaire (PHQ-9 & PHQ-2): https://bit.ly/2V7IxZ3

CHAPTER 22

Insomnia

Diagnostic Considerations

- Difficulty falling asleep, waking up during the night several times or for a long time, and/or waking too early with inability to return to sleep.
- 10–20% of adults; incidence higher among women and older age groups.

Categorized as:
- Primary/secondary (if associated with physical or psychiatric comorbidities, drugs, or substance abuse).
- Chronic/acute.

Diagnostic criteria (DSM-5):
- Dissatisfaction with sleep quantity/quality, associated with one of the following difficulty initiating/maintaining sleep, frequent awakenings, problems returning to sleep, early morning awakening.
- Significant distress / impaired functioning.
- At least 3 nights per week, for three months.

Evaluate for Symptoms

Assess sleep and waking function, precipitating factors, comorbid illness
- Ask about sleep (what time do you go to bed / fall asleep, awakening, associated symptoms, time out of bed in the morning, usual duration of sleep, general routine).
- Pre-sleep routine, i.e. bedroom, environment, vigorous activity late in evening.
- Symptoms of obstructive sleep apnoea, e.g. heavy snoring, pauses in breathing.
- Precipitants, e.g. stimulants (caffeine, cigarettes, drugs, medicines, life events).
- Naps during daytime.
- Other sleep disorder symptoms.
- Depression.
- Parasomnias (i.e. restless sleep, leg or body twitching, leg jerking – restless leg syndrome, shaking fits, sleep walking or talking, waking up in terror).

Psychiatry Algorithms for Primary Care, First Edition. Gautam Gulati, Walter Cullen, and Brendan Kelly.
© 2021 John Wiley & Sons Ltd. Published 2021 by John Wiley & Sons Ltd.

Further Evaluation

Secondary cause:
- External stimuli e.g. noise, light, etc.
- Psychological distress (depression, anxiety etc. is the cause in 50% of cases).
- Physical symptoms, e.g. pain, heartburn, restless legs, hot flushes, sleep apnoea.
- Stimulants, e.g. alcohol, caffeine, SSRIs, beta-blockers, decongestants, diuretics, steroids, recreational drugs, etc.

Impact of sleep problems:
- Does patient feel unrefreshed / still sleepy the next day?
- Any symptoms such as headache, dry mouth, daytime sleepiness?

Investigations

- Sleep diary:
  - Record sleep pattern for 1–2 weeks to identify sleep trends, such as erratic schedules, or identify predominant sleep patterns, such as taking a long time to fall asleep, frequent awakenings, early morning awakenings, or a mixture.
  - Used as 'baseline' for management of insomnia / monitor response to treatment.
- Polysomnography (overnight sleep study).

Refer to Secondary Care

- If clinical features of condition requiring investigation in secondary care (e.g. sleep apnoea).

Treatment (non-pharmacological):

- Sleep hygiene
- Relaxation therapy (music)
- Cognitive behavioural therapy (CBT)
- Digital CBT 'apps' (e.g. 'Sleepio', 'Sleepstation').

Treatment (pharmacological):

- Benzodiazepines and Z drugs (e.g. zopiclone 3.75–7.5mg nocte, zolpidem 5–10mg nocte):
  - prescribe in a minority of cases and only for short-term intermittent use for < 1 week;
  - explain risks of tolerance, that drugs are highly addictive;
  - advise about risks of driving, operating machinery, etc.; and
  - if prescribed, it should be in conjunction with specialist help, subject to regular review and attempts to stop or reduce.

- Others: Consider melatonin (2mg modified release, trial up to 13 weeks) for primary insomnia. Sedating antihistamines (e.g. promethazine 25mg) are sometimes useful as are herbal remedies.
- Where there is comorbid severe mental illness, insomnia can direct choice of antidepressants (e.g. mirtazapine) and antipsychotics (e.g. olanzapine).

Also see algorithms for	**Commonly Prescribed Drugs**
Recommended reading	1. Winkelman JW. Insomnia. *BMJ Best Practice* (last updated November 2019) (https://bit.ly/2V6EkoC). 2. Cunnington D, & Junge M. Chronic insomnia: diagnosis and non-pharmacological management. *BMJ*. 2016;355;i5819 (https://doi.org/10.1136/bmj.i5819) 3. Davidson JR, Dickson C, & Han H. Cognitive behavioural treatment for insomnia in primary care: a systematic review of sleep outcomes. *Br J Gen Pract*. 2019;69 (686): 657–664 (https://doi.org/10.3399/bjgp19X705065). 4. Kay-Stacey M, & Attarian H. Advances in the management of chronic insomnia. *BMJ*. 2016;354:i2123 (https://doi.org/10.1136/bmj.i2123). 5. Kennedy KM, & O'Riordan J. Prescribing benzodiazepines in general practice. *Br J Gen Pract*. 2019;69 (680): 152–153 (https://doi.org/10.3399/bjgp19X701753).

Resources

Benzodiazepines and Z Drugs: https://bit.ly/34s8WoV
Sleep diary, Patient.info: https://bit.ly/34fn8kZ
Sleep hygiene, Sleep Foundation: https://bit.ly/2JLUP4g
Ten tips to beat insomnia, NHS: https://bit.ly/2yFMGvO

CHAPTER 23

Medically Unexplained Symptoms

Diagnostic Considerations

Medically unexplained symptoms (MUS) and somatic symptom disorders (SSD):
- MUS can be evident in 20–45% of GP consultations.
- MUS refer to 'Persistent bodily complaints for which adequate examination (including investigation) does not reveal sufficiently explanatory structural or other specified pathology'.
- MUS are not necessarily abnormal. Many exhibit it but seldom or never seek care. MUS becomes a medical issue when it leads to healthcare-seeking for feared but non-existent physical illness and the cause of functional impairment.
- MUS can be diagnosed only by excluding organic diseases.
- In the *Diagnostic and Statistical Manual of Mental Disorders, Fourth Edition, text revised (DSM-IV-TR)* the presence of MUS was a criterion for the diagnosis of a somatic symptom disorder. In the fifth edition, DSM-5, somatoform disorders were replaced by the **somatic symptom disorder (SSD)**, consisting of a new set of criteria including psychological ones.

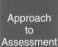

Approach to Assessment

- Acknowledge that the patient is suffering, take their concerns seriously and explore them fully, be aware of cues that suggest distress.
- Rule out medical causes but do not investigate/refer endlessly.
- Consider that there may be explanation for the symptoms but not in medical terms – rather, in terms of psychodynamic account of mental functioning.
- Consider associated depression/anxiety.
- Discuss likelihood of investigations being normal, to prevent the patient being disappointed that 'nothing has been found'.
- Focus on managing symptoms, not finding a cure.
- Consider regular planned reviews, using double appointments if needed.
- Ensure good communication with other agencies and healthcare professionals.
- Remain aware of transference (i.e. that the symptoms are being addressed to you as practitioner demanding a response) and countertransference (i.e. feelings of anger and frustration).

Psychiatry Algorithms for Primary Care, First Edition. Gautam Gulati, Walter Cullen, and Brendan Kelly.
© 2021 John Wiley & Sons Ltd. Published 2021 by John Wiley & Sons Ltd.

Somatic symptom disorders (SSD)

Presenting features:

- Unconventional behaviour during history.
- Presentation vague, dramatic, or odd.
- Problems processing emotions.
- Alexithymia (difficulty describing feelings).
- Recent/remote life stressors.
- History of childhood trauma.
- Multiple illness behaviours.
- Distractible symptoms and inconsistent examination findings.
- Unusual neurological deficits, 'give way' weakness, false sensory findings, inconsistent paralysis, bizarre movements, pseudoclonus.
- Cognitive symptoms (forgetting conversations, using wrong words, forgetting how to do basic tasks / multitask, and short-term memory problems).
- Aphonia, dysphonia, stuttering, globus hystericus.

Diagnostic criteria:

- One or more physical symptoms that are distressing or cause disruption in daily life.
- Excessive thoughts, feelings, or behaviours related to the physical symptoms or health concerns with at least one of the following: ongoing thoughts that are out of proportion with the seriousness of symptoms; ongoing high level of anxiety about health or symptoms; excessive time and energy spent on the symptoms or health concerns.
- At least one symptom is constantly present, although there may be different symptoms and symptoms may come and go (Diagnostic consideration – six months).

Subsets of SSD:

- Factitious disorder (falsification of physical or psychological signs or symptoms, or induction of injury or disease, associated with identified deception) – to the self, or by proxy.
- Illness anxiety disorder (preoccupation with having or acquiring a serious illness); somatoform disorder not otherwise specified.
- Conversion disorder (one or more symptoms of altered voluntary motor or sensory function, clinical findings provide evidence of incompatibility, symptoms not better explained by another medical or mental disorder, causing clinically significant distress or impairment).
- Psychological factors affecting other medical conditions (a medical condition must exist and psychological factors must negatively affect the condition).
- Other/unspecified SSD.

Evaluation of somatic symptom disorders:

- Evaluate for functional impairment.
- Evaluate comorbid psychiatric disorders (e.g. mood disorders, panic disorder, GAD, PTSD, dissociative disorders, social or specific phobias, OCD, personality disorders).
- At initial presentation, all patients should have laboratory testing to rule out medical or neurological conditions.

Treatment of somatic symptom disorders:

- Psychotherapy (including CBT, mindfulness, and/or psychodynamic psychotherapy).
- Psychiatric Consultation Intervention.
- Graded exercise.
- Biofeedback.
- Pharmacological treatment options for comorbid depression or anxiety include SSRIs (particularly anxiety disorders), SNRIs (particularly with predominant pain), tricyclic antidepressants, mirtazapine.
- Self-care.

Also see algorithms for	**Depression** **Generalised Anxiety Disorder** **Personality Disorders**
Recommended reading	1. Royal College of General Practitioners, Top ten tips for medically unexplained symptoms (2018) (https://bit.ly/3jHJK4L). 2. Olde Hartman TC, Lam CLK, & Usta J et al. Addressing the needs of patients with medically unexplained symptoms: 10 key messages. *Br J Gen Pract*. 2018;68 (674): 442–443 (https://doi.org/10.3399/bjgp18X698813). 3. Chew-Graham CA, Heyland S, & Kingstone T et al. Medically unexplained symptoms: continuing challenges for primary care. *Br J Gen Pract*. 2017;67 (656): 106–107 (https://doi.org/10.3399/bjgp17X689473). 4. Edwards TM, Stern A, & Clarke DD. The treatment of patients with medically unexplained symptoms in primary care: a review of the literature. *Ment Health Fam Med*. 2010 Dec; 7(4):209–221.

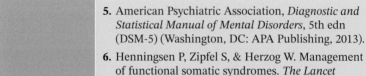

5. American Psychiatric Association, *Diagnostic and Statistical Manual of Mental Disorders*, 5th edn (DSM-5) (Washington, DC: APA Publishing, 2013).
6. Henningsen P, Zipfel S, & Herzog W. Management of functional somatic syndromes. *The Lancet* 369;9565 (2007): 946–955 (https://doi.org/10.1016/S0140-6736(07)60159-7).
7. Stonnington C, River-Dunckley E, Noe KH, & Locke D. Conversion and somatic symptom disorders. *BMJ Best Practice* (2018) (https://bit.ly/39Ra0U2).
8. Kurlansik SL, & Maffei MS. Somatic symptom disorder. *Am Fam Physician*. 2016 Jan 1; 93(1), 49–54A (https://bit.ly/2ynDLPs).

Resources

Functional Neurological Disorder (FND) – a patient's guide: https://bit.ly/2xTsKVN
PHQ-15 Somatic Symptom Severity Scale: https://bit.ly/2VlS8g0
Somatic symptom disorder, Patient.info: https://bit.ly/3e09GWz

PART 4

Complex Scenarios

CHAPTER 24

Suicide and Self Harm

Key Facts
- Globally, 800,000 people die by suicide each year; many more engage in non-fatal self-harm.
- The global rate of suicide fell by a third between 1990 and 2016.
- Suicide is the foremost cause of death worldwide in people aged between 15 and 24 years.
- Suicide is a statically rare event and so **cannot be predicted** in any individual case.

Risk Factors
- *Gender:* Suicide is more common in males; non-fatal self-harm is more common in females.
- *Specific disorders:* Depression, bipolar disorder, schizophrenia, substance misuse, epilepsy, and traumatic brain injury increase the odds of suicide by a factor greater than three.
- *Other risk factors:* Previous suicide attempt, sexual abuse in childhood, family history of suicidal behavior, and the death of a parent by suicide in early childhood.
- *Other relevant factors:* Genetics, epigenetics, early life adversity, personality disorders, physical health problems, lack of social support, economic adversity, life events, effects of the media, and access to lethal means (e.g. paracetamol tablets, high bridges).

Investigations
- *Full history*, asking especially for recent stressors, previous depression or self-harm, substance misuse, or any family history of mental illness or suicidality.
- *Collateral history*, from family, friends, or others, focusing especially on potential sources of support during a suicidal crisis.
- *Physical examination*, with particular emphasis on evidence of self-harm (e.g. self-cutting) or physical signs of mental illness (e.g. weight loss in depression, signs of anorexia nervosa).
- *Mental state examination*, with particular emphasis on mood, depressive cognitions, hopelessness, helplessness, suicidality, insight, and willingness to engage in treatment.
- *Physical investigations*, especially investigations relevant to depression (e.g. thyroid function tests) and any investigations indicated following self-harm (e.g. overdosing, self-cutting).
- *Drug testing, as indicated*, for alcohol, illegal drugs, and any other drugs of abuse.

Psychiatry Algorithms for Primary Care, First Edition. Gautam Gulati, Walter Cullen, and Brendan Kelly.
© 2021 John Wiley & Sons Ltd. Published 2021 by John Wiley & Sons Ltd.

Referral to Secondary Care

- Specialist secondary care is usually required for suicidality and self-harm, although much ongoing management and monitoring is provided in primary care and by other services.
- Refer also for severe depression, psychosis, treatment resistance, or failure of outpatient care.

Key actions	
Talking to someone who is suicidal or has self-harmed	<ul><li>**Always listen**: this person might be talking to you *instead of killing themselves.*</li><li>**Containment**: Remain calm no matter how distressed the person is; this demonstrates that the feelings that overwhelm them do *not* overwhelm you.</li><li>If you think that someone might be suicidal, but you are not certain, **ask them directly**; this does *not* increase risk and does *not* 'put the idea into their head'; if anything, it takes it out.</li><li>Ask a question along the following lines in a sympathetic but direct, matter-of-fact way: **'Are there times when you feel so low that you feel like you can't carry on? That you want to end your life, or kill yourself?'**</li><li>Most people are **hugely relieved** to talk about such distressing thoughts with someone who has the capacity to listen and not be overwhelmed by what is said.</li><li>Mostly listen. **Resist the impulse to speak** every time there is a silence.</li><li>The most important thing that you are doing is **being there**.</li><li>**Avoid platitude**s. For example, do not say: 'Don't worry. Everything is OK.' Clearly, everything is *not* OK. Saying that everything is OK just shows that you are not listening.</li><li>After a while, make one or two **very pragmatic, very short-term suggestions** (e.g. 'Why not phone your sister and see if you can call around today?'); avoid long-term suggestions (e.g. 'Why not leave your husband?'); long-term suggestions are for another day (if ever).</li><li>Remain calm, pragmatic, and hopeful as you speak and make an **immediate plan of action**.</li></ul>

Questions to ask about suicidality	• How long has the person had suicidal thoughts? Are these thoughts new or long-standing?
	• Do the suicidal thoughts wax and wane? If so, why? Is there any pattern?
	• Are there any triggers for the present suicidal crisis? Can these be addressed?
	• If suicidality is long-standing, what considerations usually stop the person from self-harming?
	• Has the person made any final acts (e.g. writing notes, saying goodbye, settling affairs)?
	• If the person has attempted self-harm, how did they come to medical attention? Did they seek medical attention themselves or were they found by chance by family or friends?
	• How does the person feel now? Are they sorry for their suicidal thoughts or acts, or sorry that they are still alive? Ambivalence is common; there is rarely a clear answer to this question.
Immediate actions in suicidality	• If the person has already taken steps to end their life, it is important that they receive medical attention, possibly at an emergency department in a hospital.
	• If the person has not taken steps to end their life but remains suicidal, it is important that means of self-harm (e.g. tablets) are removed from their immediate vicinity and that someone (e.g. a family member) is with them to support them.
	• Assist the person in accessing relevant local support services (see 'Resources', below).
	• In more acute situations, most large and regional hospitals have psychiatry services operating 24 hours a day, 7 days a week, 365 days a year, for emergency assessments.
	• It is important to remain calm and supportive at all times, and to really listen to what is being said. By confiding in you, the person has placed you in a very privileged, responsible position.
	• While you might have had many conversations with suicidal patients, this might be the first time that this patient has had such a conversation, so it might be new to them and their family.

Also see algorithms for	**Depression**
Recommended reading	1. Fazel S, & Runeson B. Suicide. *N Engl J Med* 2020; 382(1078): 266–274 (https://doi.org/10.1056/NEJMx200005). 2. Kelly BD. Suicide. *Irish Medical Journal* (in press). 3. Naghavi M, on behalf of the Global Burden of Disease Self-Harm Collaborators. Global, regional, and national burden of suicide mortality 1990 to 2016: systematic analysis for the Global Burden of Disease Study 2016. *BMJ.* 2019;364: 194 (https://doi.org/10.1136/bmj.l94).

Resources

Mind: www.mind.org.uk
NHS website: www.nhs.uk/conditions/suicide
The Samaritans: www.samaritans.org

CHAPTER 25

Aggression

Prevention

It is possible aggression (physical and verbal) can be prevented by:
- Maintaining clear therapeutic boundaries.
- Displays of a zero-tolerance policy.
- Maintaining an awareness of patients risk profiles before and during consultation.
- Staff training.
- Having risk assessments around managing patients with a known history of aggression.

Think Ahead

- Personal safety measures may include: personal alarms, consultation rooms with two exits, sitting closer to an exit, a policy of not seeing people who have a history of aggression alone and consideration to having security staff in the practice if working in a particularly vulnerable area.
- Having agreed a safety strategy beforehand, including giving thought to how to manage rare serious incidents can be beneficial. Those working in rural or vulnerable locations may have an agreement with local police.
- If a patient has a history of carrying weapons, it is worth asking for these. For the practice with security staff, screening for these is helpful.
- Extra caution is needed for domiciliary visits to those with a history of aggression. Lone working is inadvisable in these circumstances.

Causes of Aggression

- Drug or alcohol intoxication or withdrawal.
- Personality disorder (particularly antisocial but also narcissistic and borderline).
- Acute psychosis.
- Mania.
- Agitation in delirium.
- Behavioural symptoms of dementia.
- No mental disorder.

Immediate Management

- **Step 1:** Make yourself (and anyone around) safe. Run if necessary.
- **Step 2:** Call for help / raise the alarm / ask for the police if necessary.
- **Step 3:** Consider verbal de-escalation (offering space, reassurance) if appropriate.
- **Step 4:** Think as to which of the above diagnoses is likely.
- **Step 5:** Consider specialist care if appropriate. This may need involvement of police in some cases.

Psychiatry Algorithms for Primary Care, First Edition. Gautam Gulati, Walter Cullen, and Brendan Kelly.
© 2021 John Wiley & Sons Ltd. Published 2021 by John Wiley & Sons Ltd.

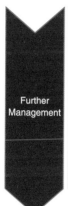

Further Management

- **Drug or alcohol intoxication or withdrawal:** Referral to the emergency department for detoxification or advise the police general practitioner if taken into custody.
- **Personality disorder:** Request advice from secondary care mental health as to how to proceed (services differ in countries). Involvement of police may have a deterrent effect on future behaviour.
- **Acute psychosis or mania:** Often need referral to secondary care mental health, sometimes using involuntary admission procedures. The use of a sedative antipsychotic such as olanzapine (oral) 5–10 mg or a benzodiazepine such as lorazepam (oral) 1–2 mg may assist the immediate situation subject to the availability of safety measures.
- **Delirium/Dementia:** Advice from secondary care may be necessary. For delirium, evaluation in general hospital to assess underlying cause may be necessary. First line medication for immediate management of aggression related to delirium or behavioural symptoms of dementia may include haloperidol (oral) 0.5–1 mg or quetiapine (oral) 12.5–25 mg.

Also see algorithms for	Psychosis Bipolar Affective Disorder Delirium Personality Disorders Substance Use Disorder Alchohol Use Disorder
Recommended reading	1. NICE Guideline [NG10]: Violence and aggression: short-term management in mental health, health and community settings (2015) (https://bit.ly/2AfJ7K0). 2. Wright NM, Dixon CA, & Tompkins CN. Managing violence in primary care: an evidence-based approach. *Br J Gen Pract.* 2003;53(492):557–562 (https://bit.ly/2mbWeZ7).

CHAPTER 26

Referrals for Involuntary Care

Key Facts

- Most psychiatric care is provided by primary care teams and community mental health services to voluntary outpatients who never experience involuntary care.
- Approximately 90% of episodes of inpatient psychiatric care are on a voluntary basis and these patients do not experience involuntary care.
- For the minority of patients who experience involuntary care, such care is closely governed by legislation owing to both (a) the requirement for involuntary treatment for people with severe mental illness who lack insight, and (b) the implications of involuntary care for various human rights including the right to liberty.

Before Considering Involuntary Care

- Like all medical care, psychiatric care should be provided on a voluntary basis whenever possible.
- Home-based treatment, community treatment, and other forms of voluntary care that are available should be comprehensively tried before involuntary psychiatric care is considered.
- Involuntary care should be used only (a) as a last resort; (b) when absolutely necessary; (c) when other, less intrusive approaches have failed; (d) for the shortest period possible; and (e) in accordance with local legislation, regulations, codes of practice, and the principles of medical ethics.
- Involuntary patients still possess all the same human rights as everyone else, albeit that specific rights, such as the right to liberty, are not observed, in part or in full, during the period of involuntary care.
- All other rights must be observed in full and any infringement on specific rights must be as limited, as brief, and as closely monitored as possible.

Psychiatry Algorithms for Primary Care, First Edition. Gautam Gulati, Walter Cullen, and Brendan Kelly.
© 2021 John Wiley & Sons Ltd. Published 2021 by John Wiley & Sons Ltd.

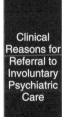

Clinical Reasons for Referral to Involuntary Psychiatric Care

- Schizophrenia and mood disorders are the psychiatric conditions most commonly associated with involuntary psychiatric care.
- Common clinical reasons for referral for consideration for involuntary psychiatric care in various jurisdictions include: (a) severe symptoms, especially psychosis, with lack of insight; (b) treatment resistance; (c) perceived risk of suicide, self-harm, or self-neglect; (d) perceived risk of harm to others; (e) perceived risk of harm to property; (f) perceived lack of mental capacity or decision-making capacity in relation to mental health care; (g) failure of outpatient care in certain cases; and (h) referral by various elements of the criminal justice system (e.g. police services, judges).
- The initial decision about referral for consideration for involuntary care should be a clinical one, regardless of the legal or judicial arrangements in any given jurisdiction; subsequent reviews may be somewhat legal or judicial in nature, but they should remain focused on the severity and urgency of the patient's clinical needs.
- When assessing someone for involuntary care, it is generally best to explain clearly and directly what is going on; in the rare, extreme cases where such openness is judged to be inadvisable in terms of patient well-being, explanations should be provided as soon as feasible.
- For the most part, clear, direct communication is best from the outset; while such clear communication might cause conflict at the time, it minimises subsequent problems and results in a much better doctor–patient relationship in the longer term.

After Involuntary Care

- Reactions to involuntary care vary greatly; a significant proportion of recovered patients are grateful for their involuntary care, but a significant proportion find the experience traumatic.
- In primary care, it is important to both (a) maintain a good long-term relationship with the patient and their family, and (b) acknowledge the reality of the involuntary admission process, in which the general practitioner might have played a role, depending on the jurisdiction.
- Following involuntary psychiatric care, the great majority of patients will require ongoing treatment and management in primary care, in partnership with their community mental health team.

Legal criteria for involuntary psychiatric care

- Legal criteria for involuntary psychiatric care vary across jurisdictions but usually involve various combinations of four key concepts: (i) mental disorder; (ii) risk to self or others; (iii) need for treatment; and (iv) mental capacity or decision-making capacity in relation to mental health care.
- Definitions of mental disorder vary greatly across jurisdictions, but such definitions are central elements of criteria for involuntary care in most countries: for example, in England and Wales the Mental Health Act 1983 defines 'mental disorder' as 'any disorder or disability of the mind' (a very broad definition).

- Risk to self and others is difficult or impossible to quantify, but it nonetheless features in criteria for involuntary psychiatric care in many countries: for example, in England and Wales the criteria for involuntary 'admission for assessment' include that the person 'ought to be so detained in the interests of his own health or safety or with a view to the protection of other persons'; and criteria for involuntary 'admission for treatment' include that such treatment 'is necessary for the health or safety of the patient or for the protection of other persons'.

- A need for treatment and likelihood of benefit are also criteria for involuntary care in many jurisdictions: for example, in England and Wales the criteria for involuntary 'admission for treatment' include that 'it is necessary for the health or safety of the patient or for the protection of other persons that he should receive such treatment and it cannot be provided unless he is detained under this section', and that 'appropriate medical treatment is available'.

- Certain jurisdictions include a mental capacity (or decision-making capacity) test in their criteria for involuntary psychiatric care, generally requiring that the person lacks the ability to make their own decisions about psychiatric care if involuntary care is to be considered. Key elements of mental capacity are abilities to: (i) understand relevant information; (ii) retain the information for long enough to make a decision; (iii) use or weigh the information; and (iv) communicate the decision.

Also see algorithms for	**Depression** **Psychosis** **Self-Harm and Suicide**
Recommended reading	**1.** Cockburn P, & Cockburn H, *Henry's Demons: Living with Schizophrenia; A Father and Son's Story* (London: Simon & Schuster, 2011).
	2. Feeney A, Umama-Agada E, Gilhooley J et al. Gender, diagnosis and involuntary psychiatry admission in Ireland: a report from the Dublin Involuntary Admission Study (DIAS). *International Journal of Law and Psychiatry* 2019; 66:101472 (https://doi.org/10.1016/j.ijlp.2019.101472).
	3. Szmukler G, *Men in White Coats: Treatment Under Coercion* (Oxford: Oxford University Press, 2018).
	4. Zigmond T, *A Clinician's Brief Guide to the Mental Health Act*, 3rd edn (London: RCPsych Publications, 2014).

Resources

Mental Health Commmission Guide (Ireland): https://www.mhcirl.ie/file/refguidmha2001p1.pdf

Mind: http://www.mind.org.uk/information-support/legal-rights/sectioning/overview

NHS: https://www.nhs.uk/using-the-nhs/nhs-services/mental-health-services/mental-health-act

PART 5

Special Considerations In Prescribing

CHAPTER 27

Special Considerations: Older Adults

General Principles

- Avoid psychotropic medication if at all possible. Psychosocial approaches are preferable.
- Use low doses where medication is needed (often half the adult starting dose*).
- Titrate doses slowly.
- Monitor for response frequently.
- Avoid polypharmacy.
- Avoid adding new medication to treat side effects – try something different that is tolerated better.

*Refer to an up-to-date guideline and summary of product characteristics (SPC) for medication.

Secondary Care

- Request secondary care advice early. Particularly with psychotic symptoms, suspicion of underlying cognitive impairment, safeguarding concerns, complex issues around capacity, or in the case of depression where first line treatment has not worked or there is prominent suicidal ideation. This is a specialist area.
- Loss of appetite and weight loss are concerning symptoms but may need initial referral to a geriatrician.
- New onset bipolar affective disorder is uncommon in the elderly. Investigate for an underlying physical cause first.

Key Considerations

Use these six questions as a guide before prescribing:
1. Is this medication absolutely necessary? Are there alternatives?
2. Which is the agent and dose that best combines safety with tolerability?
3. Will this medication interact with anything else that is prescribed?
4. Will this medication affect any existing physical illness (particularly ophthalmic, neurological, gastrointestinal, cardiovascular, pulmonary)?
5. Is there existing hepatic or renal impairment that needs to be taken into consideration?
6. Are there any aspects of the receptor profile of the drug that means it will likely be a problem for this patient? Such as constipation or urinary retention with anticholinergics, hypotension and falls with alpha blockers.

Psychiatry Algorithms for Primary Care, First Edition. Gautam Gulati, Walter Cullen, and Brendan Kelly.
© 2021 John Wiley & Sons Ltd. Published 2021 by John Wiley & Sons Ltd.

Consent

- There is a presumption of capacity to consent.
- In the absence of capacity, proceed as with the legal requirements in your jurisdiction.
- General principles in patients lacking decision making capacity include:
  - Advance directives should be respected.
  - Considering the best interests of the patient through consulting family, carers and professionals.
  - Covert adminstration should not be routinely used. This should only be considered with legal safeguards using mental capacity legislation in order to reduce a patient's distress.

Examples of medication choice and dosage (1st line)

	Comments	Caution
Depression		
Ideally SSRI such as sertraline starting at 25mg or citalopram 10mg	Less interactions	Hyponatremia, bleeding
Mirtazapine starting at 7.5mg nocte	May assist sleep	Sedation, constipation, urinary retention
Anxiety		
SSRI such as sertraline starting at 25mg or citalopram 10mg		Hyponatremia, bleeding
Acute mania or psychosis		
Quetiapine starting at 12.5–25mg BD		Monitor for sedation and postural hypotension. Increased risk of stroke in patients with dementia
Risperidone starting at 0.5mg		Monitor for increased prolactin. Increased risk of stroke in patients with dementia
Aripiprazole starting at 5mg		Monitor for agitation
Agitation		
Clonazepam starting at 0.5mg		Sedatives can worsen confusion, and carry a higher risk of respiratory depression in the elderly

Insomnia		
Zopiclone starting at 3.75mg	Trial not to exceed 4 weeks	Can worsen confusion

Also see algorithms for	**Delirium** **Dementia**
Recommended reading	1. Taylor DM, Barnes TRE, & Young AH, *The Maudsley Prescribing Guidelines in Psychiatry*, 13th edn (Hoboken, NJ; Chichester, UK: Wiley, 2018).
	2. NHS England and NHS Improvement, *Mental Health in Older People: A Practice Primer* (2017) (https://bit.ly/2lTnueP).

CHAPTER 28

Special Considerations in Prescribing: Children and Adolescents

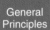

General Principles

- Diagnoses should be made with caution and keeping in context the child's developmental age.
- Psychological approaches are first line treatments. Where medication is used, this should be in combination with psychosocial treatment.
- Where medication is used*:
  - Titrate doses slowly, monitor for response frequently, avoid polypharmacy unless in consultation with secondary care.
  - Always include parents/carers in decision-making.
  - Clearly document indication, rationale, and (parental) consent if using an off-label medication.

*refer to an uptodate guideline and Summary of Product Characteristics (SPC) for medication

Secondary Care

- Request secondary care advice early. Particularly with psychotic symptoms, suspicion of bipolar disorder, child protection concerns, or in the case of depression where first line treatment has not worked or there is prominent suicidal ideation. This is a specialist area.
- Referral is to Child and Adolescent Mental Health Services (CAMHS). A referral to paediatrics may be helpful with suspected neurodevelopmental conditions. In some areas, early intervention in psychosis teams assess patients with suspected psychosis older than 14 years.

Psychiatry Algorithms for Primary Care, First Edition. Gautam Gulati, Walter Cullen, and Brendan Kelly.
© 2021 John Wiley & Sons Ltd. Published 2021 by John Wiley & Sons Ltd.

Medication used in children and adolescents (check licence in your jurisdiction)

Indication	Caution
Depression Fluoxetine starting at 5–10mg is licensed in some jurisdictions for 8–18 years. Escitalopram starting at 5mg is licensed in some jurisdictions (Trial duration 4–6 weeks)	Medication must be used only in conjunction with psychological and social interventions and only in moderate-severe cases. Psychological treatments are first line in less severe cases With any SSRI, monitor for emergence of agitation and suicidal ideation
Anxiety Sertraline starting at 12.5–25mg (Trial duration 6–8 weeks)	Medication use is second line to psychological treatment. It is used where psychological input has not worked or the young person is so severely disabled by anxiety that symptoms preclude psychological intervention With any SSRI, monitor for emergence of agitation and suicidal ideation
OCD Sertraline starting at 12.5–25mg is licensed in some jurisdictions for age >6 years. Fluvoxamine is licensed in other jurisdictions (Trial duration 12 weeks)	Medication use is second line to CBT With any SSRI, monitor for emergence of agitation and suicidal ideation
Acute mania or psychosis Aripiprazole starting at 2mg OR Olanzapine starting at 5mg OR Risperidone starting at 0.5mg (Trial duration 3–5 weeks)	Monitor for extrapyramidal symptoms, sedation, and weight gain. Blood tests (metabolic profile and prolactin) needed at baseline, 3 months and 6-monthly. Monitor height, weight, hip circumference, nutritional status

ADHD	
Methylphenidate, dexamfetamine, lisdexamfetamine, atomoxetine and guanfacine are used – however these are always initiated by secondary care	Psychosocial and behavioural treatments are first line for mild to moderate ADHD. Medication is used first line in severe cases. Diagnosis and initiation of medication should be in secondary care. Primary care may need to monitor height, weight, blood pressure, and heart rate
Insomnia	
Melatonin starting at 2mg (off-label)	Medication use is always second line. Secondary causes of insomnia need to be investigated and treated. There should be an adequate trial of sleep hygiene and targeted behavioural parent led interventions before a trial of medication is considered

Recommended reading	1. Taylor DM, Barnes TRE, & Young AH, *The Maudsley Prescribing Guidelines in Psychiatry*, 13th edn (Hoboken, NJ; Chichester, UK: Wiley, 2018).
	2. NICE Guideline [NG134]: Depression in children and young people (2019) (https://bit.ly/2Jb3zzW).
	3. NICE Guideline [CG155]: Psychosis and schizophrenia in children and young people (2016) (https://bit.ly/2ksHqF6).
	4. Creswell C, Waite P, & Cooper PJ. Assessment and management of anxiety disorders in children and adolescents. *Archives of Disease in Childhood* 2014; 99:674–678 (http://doi.org/10.1136/archdischild-2013-303768).

CHAPTER 29

Special Considerations in Prescribing: People with Intellectual Disabilities

Is Medication Necessary?

- Do not use psychotropic medication as first line treatment for behavioural disturbance.
- Rule out physical causes; infection (especially LRTI/UTI), seizures, pain (including dental), reflux, or constipation.
- Rule out environmental changes e.g. bereavement, change of carer, new fellow resident, etc., which may have caused a behavioural change.
- Rule out sexual/physical/emotional abuse.
- Would a behavioural intervention be better?

Advice from Secondary Care

- Request secondary care **involvement in initiation** and monitoring of psychotropics. This may involve a psychiatrist specialising in intellectual disabilities and/or a neurologist.

Prescribe with Caution

- Side effects to medications are very common, even at low doses.
- Optimise existing medication in preference to combining psychotropics.
- If considering medication; start on a very low dose, escalate slowly, monitor frequently for desired response and side effects.

Care Around Syndromes

- Genetic syndromes, when present may carry physical health risks, e.g. Down's Syndrome and/or behavioural phenotypes, e.g. Prader Willi.
- Consider known cardiac, neurological, ophthalmic, endocrinal, and gastrointestinal components of any underlying syndrome.

Psychiatry Algorithms for Primary Care, First Edition. Gautam Gulati, Walter Cullen, and Brendan Kelly.
© 2021 John Wiley & Sons Ltd. Published 2021 by John Wiley & Sons Ltd.

Epilepsy
- Comorbid seizure disorder is common, can be unrecognised and when present, easily destabilised.
- Seek specialist advice early as most psychotropics reduce seizure thresholds.
- Seek advice from a neurologist if in doubt.

Consent
- Careful consideration needs to be given around capacity and consent; there is a presumption of capacity and autonomy around healthcare decision-making should be respected and encouraged with support as necessary.
- Involve professionals, advocates, and family with knowledge of the patient who can contribute to 'best interests' decisions if this becomes necessary.

Also see algorithms for	**Autism Spectrum Disorder**
Recommended reading	1. Bhaumik S, Gangadharan SK, Branford D, & Barrett M, *The Frith Prescribing Guidelines for People with Intellectual Disability*, 3rd edn (Oxford: Wiley-Blackwell, 2015).
	2. Royal College of Psychiatrists, *Challenging Behaviour: A Unified Approach* (London: RCP, 2007) (https://bit.ly/2FRfvGw).
	3. Shankar R, & Wilcock M. Improving knowledge of psychotropic prescribing in people with Intellectual Disability in primary care. *PLoS One.* 2018;13(9):e0204178 (https://bit.ly/2ZnVbaA).
	4. NICE Guideline [NG11]: Challenging behaviour and learning disabilities (2015) (https://bit.ly/3esDfz1).

CHAPTER 30

Special Considerations in Prescribing: Pregnancy and Breastfeeding

General Principles

- No medication is completely safe. Some medications have more safety data than others.
- The first trimester is most risky in terms of congenital malformation risk.
- New onset non-severe illness can often be treated with non-pharmacological means.
- The use of medication is a risk–benefit decision made in conjunction with the patient.
- For existing illness, abrupt discontinuation is often unwise.
- For existing illness, staying with a medication that is working is often wiser than switching.
- Medication carries risk, but so does untreated severe mental illness.
- Always refer to an up-to-date guideline and summary of product characteristics (SPC) for medication.

Advice from Secondary Care

- Request secondary care advice as necessary. Particularly with severe mental illness such as moderate/severe depression, bipolar affective disorder, and psychotic disorders. This is a specialist area and if you have access to a specialist in Perinatal Psychiatry, they would be the best source of advice.

Pre-Pregnancy

- The best time to discuss medication is whilst planning a pregnancy.
- This may require stopping antipsychotics that elevate prolactin as these may affect fertility as well as stopping known teratogens like sodium valproate.
- Counselling should include clearly documented and jointly made risk–benefit decisions. For example, in someone whith numerous severe relapses where they have become a risk to themselves or others, remaining on an effective medication may carry greater weight than in someone who has a history of uncomplicated single episode illness.

Psychiatry Algorithms for Primary Care, First Edition. Gautam Gulati, Walter Cullen, and Brendan Kelly.
© 2021 John Wiley & Sons Ltd. Published 2021 by John Wiley & Sons Ltd.

In Pregnancy

- **Depression:** SSRI's e.g. sertraline (except paroxetine which is a known teratogen) appear not to be major teratogens. Obstetrician should be informed to monitor for hypertension, pre-eclampsia, and post partum haemorrhage. Neonatologist should be advised in advance of delivery.
- **Psychosis:** Olanzapine, risperidone, quetiapine are unlikely to be major teratogens. Obstetrician should be informed to monitor for gestational diabetes. Neonatologist should be advised in advance of delivery.
- **Bipolar disorder:** Use atypical antipsychotics as mood stabilisers where necessary as most mood stabilisers and particularly sodium valproate, lithium and carbamazepine are known teratogens. Inform obstetrician and neonatologist.
- Avoid benzodiazepines.

Breast Feeding

- The decision for breast vs bottle feeding is person centered and a risk–benefit discussion; however, advise against breastfeeding on clozapine and lithium.
- The drug used during pregnancy is often the best choice as post-partum is a high-risk time for relapse.
- If initiating a new medication, sertraline for depression and olanzapine for psychosis or mania are relatively better choices. It is best to avoid benzodiazepines.
- Consult/inform the neonatologist.

Recommended reading

1. Taylor DM, Barnes TRE, & Young AH, *The Maudsley Prescribing Guidelines in Psychiatry,* 13th edn (Hoboken, NJ; Chichester, UK: Wiley, 2018).

2. Jones I, Chandra PS, Dazzan P, & Howard LM. Bipolar disorder, affective psychosis and schizophrenia in pregnancy and the post-partum period. *The Lancet,* 384(9956), 1789–1799 (2014) (https://doi.org/10.1016/S0140-6736(14)61278-2).

3. NICE Clinical guideline [CG192]: Antenatal and postnatal mental health: clinical management and service guidance (last updated Feb 2020) (https://bit.ly/1GGNRTP).

PART 6

Appendices

CHAPTER 31

Commonly Prescribed Drugs

Psychiatry Algorithms for Primary Care, First Edition. Gautam Gulati,
Walter Cullen, and Brendan Kelly.
© 2021 John Wiley & Sons Ltd. Published 2021 by John Wiley & Sons Ltd.

Psychotropic (in alphabetical order)	Indication	Prescribing (adult dosage advice)[a]	Common side effects	Stopping treatment
Alprazolam	Short-term use in anxiety	250–500mcg 3 times a day, increase to 3mg daily	Appetite changes, impaired concentration, constipation, disorientation, dry mouth, hypersomnia, lethargy, memory loss, nervousness, sexual dysfunction, blurred vision	Care needed around development of psychological and physical dependence; a withdrawal syndrome may occur on abrupt cessation after long-term use
Amitriptyline	Major depression[b]	Initially 50mg daily in 2 doses, then increase in steps of 25mg daily on alternate days if required to maximum dose 150mg daily (in 2 doses)	Anticholinergic syndrome, drowsiness, QT interval prolongation	
Citalopram	Depressive illness	20mg once daily increasing at intervals of 3–4 weeks to maximum 40mg daily	Acute glaucoma, apathy, flatulence, hypersalivation, migraine, rhinitis	Reduce dose gradually over 4 weeks or longer if withdrawal symptoms emerge (over 6 months if long-term treatment)
	Panic disorder	Initially 10mg daily increasing in steps of 10mg daily; usual dose 20–30mg daily; maximum dose 40mg daily		

Drug	Indication	Dose	Side effects	Cautions
Diazepam[c]	Anxiety	2mg three times daily, increasing to 15–30mg daily	Appetite problems, movement, muscle spasms, palpitations, sensory disorders	Care needed around development of psychological and physical dependence; a withdrawal syndrome may occur on abrupt cessation after long-term use
	Insomnia associated with anxiety	5–15mg nocte		
	Severe acute anxiety / control of panic attacks / acute alcohol withdrawal	10mg, then 10mg after 4 hours		
Donepezil	Mild to moderate Alzheimer's dementia	5mg nocte for 1 month, increased to 10mg nocte if necessary	Aggression, agitation, appetite changes, diarrhoea, dizziness, fatigue, gastrointestinal disorders, hallucinations, headache, muscle cramps, sleep disorders, syncope, urinary incontinence, nausea and vomiting	
Duloxetine	Major depressive disorder	60mg daily	Anxiety, appetite loss, constipation, diarrhoea, dizziness, dry mouth, falls, fatigue, flushing, GI discomfort, headache paraesthesia, sexual dysfunction, sleep disorders, sweating	Reduce dose over 1–2 weeks and monitor for withdrawal changes
	Generalised anxiety disorder	Initially 30mg daily, increase if necessary to 60mg daily to a maximum of 120mg daily		

Fluoxetine	Major depression Obsessive compulsive disorder	Initially 20mg daily, increase dose if necessary after 3–4 weeks; with insufficient response to 20mg, dose may be increased gradually up to 60mg on an individual patient basis, to maintain patients at the lowest effective dose	Gastrointestinal disturbance, anxiety, agitation, nausea, weight loss, chills, haemorrhage, postmenopausal bleeding, blurred vision, uterine disorder; vasodilation	
	Bulimia nervosa	60mg daily		
Memantine	Moderate to severe dementia	Initially 5mg daily, increase in steps of 5mg every week to usual maintenance of 20mg daily	Impaired balance, constipation, dizziness, drowsiness, dyspnoea, headache, hypersensitivity, hypertension	
Mirtazapine	Major depression	Initially 15–30mg daily for 2–4 weeks, at bedtime; adjust according to response to 45mg daily (as single or 2 doses)	Anxiety, appetite increase, arthralgia, back pain, confusion, constipation diarrhoea, dizziness, drowsiness, dry mouth, fatigue, headaches (on discontinuation), myalgia, nausea, oedema, postural hypotension, sleep disorders, tremor, vomiting, weight gain	Dose should be reduced over several weeks

Olanzapine	Schizophrenia	10mg daily, adjust according to response; maximum dose 20mg daily	Sedation, increased appetite, arthralgia, oedema, anticholinergic syndrome, asthenia, drowsiness, eosinophilia, fever, glycosuria, hypersomnia, postural hypotension, dyslipidemia, malaise	
	Preventing recurrence in bipolar disorder			
	Mania	15mg daily, adjust according to response; maximum dose 20mg daily		
	Control of agitation and disturbed behaviour in schizophrenia / mania	(IM) Initially 5–10mg for 1 dose, followed by 5–10mg after 2 hours if required		
Pregabalin	Generalised anxiety disorder[d]	Initially 150mg daily in 2–3 doses then increase in steps of 150mg daily if required, dose to be increased at seven-day intervals up to 600mg daily in 2–3 doses	Abdominal distension, appetite abnormalities, asthenia, concentration impaired, confusion, constipation, diarrhoea, dizziness, drowsiness, dry mouth, gastrointestinal disorders, headache, altered mood, movement disorders, muscle complaints, nausea, oedema, sexual dysfunction, sleep disorders	Avoid stopping abruptly, taper over at least 1 week

| Quetiapine | Schizophrenia | (Immediate release) 25mg twice daily for day 1, then 50mgs twice daily for day 2, then 100mg twice daily for day 3, then 150mg twice daily for day 3, then adjust to response to usual dose 300–450mg daily in divided doses and maximum dose 750mg daily.

(Modified release) 300mg once daily for day 1, then 600mg once daily for day 2, then adjust to response to usual dose 600mg daily in divided doses and maximum dose 800mg daily | Increased appetite, asthenia, dysarthria, dyspepsia, dyspnoea, fever, headache, irritability, palpitations, peripheral oedema, postural hypotension, rhinitis, sleep disorders, syncope, blurred vision |
| | Adjunctive treatment of major depression | (Modified release) 50mg daily at bedtime for 2 days, then 150mg once daily for 2 days, then adjust to response to usual dose 150–300mg daily. | |

Risperidone				
	Schizophrenia	2mg daily, increased in steps of 1mg to a maximum of 10mg/day. Unusually, higher doses may be needed, maximum 16mg/day	Sedation, increased prolactin, extrapyramidal side-effects at higher doses, anaemia, anxiety, appetite disturbance, asthenia, chest discomfort, conjunctivitis, cough, depression, diarrhoea, dyspnoea, epistaxis, fall, fever, gastrointestinal discomfort, headache, hyperglycaemia, hypertension, oedema, sexual dysfunction	
	Mania	2mg daily titrating upwards to max 6mg daily		
	Short-term treatment (up to six weeks) of persistent aggression in patients with moderate to severe Alzheimer's dementia unresponsive to non-pharmacological interventions	0.25mg bd max 0.5mg bd	ECG may be needed. Specific risks when used in the elderly – seek specialist guidance.	

Sertraline	Depressive illness Obsessive compulsive disorder	Initially 50mg daily Increase in steps of 50mg at weekly intervals to a maximum of 200mg daily	Chest pain, depression, GI disorders, vasodilation, neuromuscular dysfunction	Reduce dose gradually over 4-week period, or longer if withdrawal symptoms emerge (6 months if patient has been on long-term treatment)
	Panic disorder	Initially 25mg daily for one week, then increase to 50mg daily, then increase in steps of 50mg at weekly intervals to a maximum of 200mgs daily		
Venlafaxine	Major depression	Initially 75mg daily (as single dose if modified release or 2 doses of 37.5mg if immediate release medicines). Increase dose if necessary at intervals of 2 weeks up to 375mg daily	Anxiety, appetite change, arrhythmias, chills, asthenia, confusion, constipation, depersonalisation, diarrhoea, dizziness, dry mouth, dyspnoea, headache, hot flush, hypertension, menstrual cycle irregularities, movement disorders, muscle tone, nausea, palpitations, paraesthesia, sedation, sexual dysfunction, sweating, taste changes, tinnitus, tremor, urinary disorders, vision disorders, vomiting, weight loss, yawning	Higher risk of withdrawal effects compared to other antidepressants Reduce dose over several weeks
	Generalised anxiety disorder Social anxiety disorder	Initially 75mg daily (as single dose of modified release) Increase dose if necessary at intervals of 2 weeks up to 225mg daily		

Zolpidem	Insomnia (short-term use)	10mg daily for up to 4 weeks, dose to be taken at bedtime[e]	Abdominal pain, anterograde amnesia, anxiety, back pain, diarrhoea, dizziness, fatigue, hallucinations, headache
Zopiclone	Insomnia (short-term use)	7.5mg daily for up to 4 weeks, at bedtime	Dry mouth, anterograde amnesia, fatigue, metallic taste

Notes

[a] Note lower doses to be prescribed in the elderly, please check BNF.

[b] Not recommended in those with cardiac history as increased risk of fatality in overdose.

[c] Other indications include: muscle spasm of varied aetiology, acute muscle spasm, tetanus, muscle spasm in cerebral spasticity, acute drug inducted dystonia, premedication, sedation, status epilepticus, convulsions, dyspnoea associated with anxiety in palliative care, pain or muscle spasm in palliative care.

[d] Other indications:peripheral/central neuropathic pain, adjunctive therapy for localised seizures with secondary generalization.

[e] Use elderly dose if debilitated.

Resources

British National Formulary (2018–19) 76th edn, 2019: www.bnf.org
Health Service Executive (PCRS), The top 100 most commonly prescribed products in the order of their prescribing frequency, November, 2019: https://www.sspcrs.ie/portal/annual-reporting/report/pharmacy

CHAPTER 32

Physical Health in Patients with Severe Mental Illness

Considerations:

- Decreased life expectancy among people with psychosis (20 years for men, 15 for women) and this is due to:
  - Increased cardiometabolic risk factors (smoking, obesity, sedentary lifestyle, social deprivation) – most of the increase in mortality is due to cardiovascular/respiratory disease and cancer.
  - Antipsychotic medication increases risk via iatrogenic weight gain, hyperlipidaemia and diabetes.
  - Impaired access to healthcare and reduced uptake of screening and preventative care.
  - Increased risk of suicide, accidents, violent death.

At initiation of prescribing antipsychotic:

- Review at baseline and at least once after three months.
- Monitor weight weekly in the first 6 weeks of taking a new antipsychotic (rapid early weight gain may predict severe weight gain in the longer term).
- Subsequent reviews annually unless physical health problem emerges.

At review:

- History:
  - Substantial weight gain (e.g. 5kg), especially where this has been rapid.
  - Smoking.
  - Exercise.
  - Diet.

Psychiatry Algorithms for Primary Care, First Edition. Gautam Gulati, Walter Cullen, and Brendan Kelly.
© 2021 John Wiley & Sons Ltd. Published 2021 by John Wiley & Sons Ltd.

- Family history (diabetes, obesity, CVD in first degree relatives (< 55 years if male and < 65 years if female relative).
- Gestational diabetes.
- Ethnicity.
- Examination: Weight and waist circumference, BMI, BP, pulse.
- Investigations: Annual FBC, U&E's, LFTs, fasting plasma glucose, HbA1c, fasting lipids, prolactin.
- ECG: Especially, if history of CVD, family history of CVD, irregular pulse or if patient taking certain antipsychotics/drugs known to cause ECG abnormalities. The safest approach would be to consider at least annual ECG monitoring for every individual on long-term antipsychotics.
- Chronic kidney disease: If coexisting diabetes, hypertension, CVD, family history of chronic kidney disease, structural renal disease (e.g. renal stones) then monitor renal function.

Intervention:
- Lifestyle:
  - Nutritional counselling: Reduce take-away / 'junk' food, reduce energy intake.
  - Weight gain: Avoid soft / caffeinated drinks / juices, increase fibre intake.
  - Physical activity: Advise 30 minutes of physical activity 5 days a week.
- Pharmacological:
  - Anti-hypertensive therapy.
  - Lipid-lowering therapy.
  - Diabetes treatment.

Review of antipsychotic and mood stabiliser medication:
- Discussions about medication should involve patient, GP, and psychiatrist.
- Consider as a priority if rapid weight gain or deterioration in BP, lipids, glucose.
- Secondary care should maintain responsibility for at least the first 12 months or until the person's condition has stabilised, whichever is longer.
- Aripiprazole, quetiapine less likely to cause weight gain than olanzapine and clozapine.

Additional monitoring for clozapine and lithium

	Clozapine	Lithium
Regular monitoring	Weekly FBC for first 18 weeks, then fortnightly from week 19 to week 52, then monthly thereafter. Monitor BP, pulse and weight at each visit	Serum lithium level 5 days after initiation or dose adjustment. Sample should be taken 12 hours after last dose. Once target level of 0.6–0.8 mmol/L achieved, repeat at 3- monthly intervals. Monitor BP, pulse, and weight at each visit
6-monthly	Physical examination	Physical examination Thyroid function, renal function
Annually	Fasting plasma glucose, HbA1c, fasting lipids, FBC, U&E, LFT ECG Clozapine levels	Fasting plasma glucose, HbA1c, fasting lipids, FBC, U&E, LFT ECG
Caution	If patient cuts down or quits smoking, the clozapine dose will typically need to be reduced	Significant dehydration or drug interactions can cause lithium levels to rise to toxic levels. Hold lithium and take urgent serum lithium level

Recommended reading	1. Assessing physical health – NICE Quality standard [QS80]: Psychosis and schizophrenia in adults (https://bit.ly/2K966LS). 2. NICE Clinical guideline [CG178]: Psychosis and schizophrenia in adults: prevention and management (2014) (https://bit.ly/2Vowbf6). 3. Taylor DM, Barnes TRE, & Young AH. *The Maudsley Prescribing Guidelines in Psychiatry*, 13th edn (Hoboken, NJ; Chichester, UK: Wiley, 2018).

Resources

Shiers DE, Rafi I, Cooper SJ, & Holt RIG. *Positive Cardiometabolic Health Resource: an intervention framework for patients with psychosis and schizophrenia* (London: Royal College of Psychiatrists, 2014): https://bit.ly/2ydf6NA

PART 7

Self-Assessment

Self-Assessment Cases

The Case of Mrs A

1. You review a 33-year-old lady, Mrs A presenting with low mood, anhedonia, and a lack of energy for 4 weeks. Her appetite is poor and she has lost weight. She has been on sertraline 50mg for 2 weeks and reports only minimal benefit. Would you:

   a. Suggest a higher dose of sertraline and to give it more time

   b. Switch to amitryptiline

   c. Switch to venlafaxine

   d. Augment the antidepressant with olanzapine

   e. Refer to secondary care

2. You see Mrs A over the next few weeks. There is some improvement but still significant residual symptoms on sertraline 200mg. You decide to switch medication to escitalopram as she, on discussion, expresses a preference for something 'of the same type' which is not sedative. Would you:

   a. Stop the sertraline that day and commence escitalopram 5mg the next day

   b. Stop the Sertraline that day and commence escitalopram 20mg the next day

   c. Gradually withdraw the sertraline, stop, and then commence and up-titrate escitalopram

   d. Gradually withdraw the sertraline, stop, wait for 2 weeks and then up-titrate escitalopram

   e. Add the Escitalopram to the prescription and evaluate combination treatment

3. Mrs A still has problematic symptoms after 4 months and did not feel the escitalopram helped fully. You have referred her for counselling and she has commenced this. She is not suicidal. She is keen you do not prescribe something that will cause excessive weight gain. Would you:

   a. Switch to mirtazapine

   b. Augment with olanzapine

   c. Add lithium

   d. Switch to venlafaxine

   e. Switch to tranylcypramine

4. You decide to switch Mrs A to venlafaxine XL. Would you:

  a. Stop the escitalopram that day and commence venlafaxine XL 75mg the next day

  b. Stop the escitalopram that day and commence venlafaxine XL 225mg the next day

  c. Gradually withdraw the escitalopram, stop, and then commence and up-titrate venlafaxine

  d. Gradually withdraw the escitalopram, stop, wait for 2 weeks and then up-titrate venlafaxine

  e. Add the venlafaxine to the prescription and evaluate combination treatment

5. In which of the following circumstances would you refer Mrs A to secondary care?

  a. A failure to respond to adequate trials of two or more antidepressants

  b. Suicidal ideation with intent

  c. Psychomotor retardation and nihilistic delusions

  d. None of the above

  e. All of the above

The Case of Ms B

6. Ms B is a 19-year-old woman who has a history of panic attacks and low mood. She has never been severely depressed and never self-harmed. Her main concern was her panic attacks. These responded well to paroxetine prescribed by you. She attends your surgery on a Monday morning to report that she has missed her period and has a positive pregnancy test. She is anxious about her future. Would you:

  a. Reassure her and continue paroxetine

  b. Advise stopping the paroxetine at least for the first trimester

  c. Prescribe diazepam for anxiety

  d. Switch the paroxetine to venlafaxine

  e. Switch the paroxetine to sertraline

7. Ms B comes off her paroxetine in the first trimester and copes well without many symptoms. She consults you in the fourth month of the pregnancy with 3 weeks of low mood, anhedonia, poor energy, decreased appetite, and is withdrawing socially. She feels negative about her future and that of

her baby. You recommend psychological treatment but she does not wish to pursue this. Would you:

  a. Recommence paroxetine

  b. Wait and watch

  c. Suggest a trial of sertraline

  d. Suggest a trial of clomipramine

  e. Suggest a trial of amitryptiline

8. Ms B recovers from depression on sertraline 100mg. You inform the obstetrician and neonatologist of this prescription. She gives birth to a healthy baby girl and is discharged home. You get a call from the district nurse to ask for advice on this medication and breastfeeding as the patient is anxious about it. Do you suggest:

  a. Avoiding breastfeeding. Bottle feeding is preferable

  b. Reassuring the patient that this is a relatively safe choice in breastfeeding

  c. Stopping the sertraline immediately

  d. Taking a lower dose of sertraline

  e. A 4-week course of diazepam

9. Ms B comes to see you with her 2-month-old baby, and is feeling well. She is on sertraline 100mg. She asks how long she should continue it given that she has had only one episode of depression and now is well for 4 months. Do you advise:

  a. This can now be discontinued as she is well

  b. Continuing this for another 5–6 months before considering discontinuation

  c. Continuing this for 2 years for relapse prevention

The Case of Mr C

10. Mr C is a 42-year-old chef who presents with low mood, poor sleep, poor appetite, feeling tired, and reports feeling anxious. On evaluating his history, you discover that he is drinking three 75cl bottles of wine daily. His liver enzymes are deranged. There is a history of epilepsy and he is taking phenytoin erratically. Do you:

  a. Commence an antidepressant

  b. Prescribe a short course of benzodiazepines

  c. Refer for a psychiatric inpatient admission

  d. Refer to general hospital for detoxification

11. Mr C attends a general hospital and is discharged shortly after detoxification. His liver enzymes are still deranged. You are considering a trial of antidepressants as his mood is still low after the detoxification. Which of the following would you be least likely to prescribe?

    a. Sertraline

    b. Agomelatine

    c. Escitalopram

    d. Fluoxetine

    e. Vortioxetine

12. Mr C commences fluoxetine. He is also on prescribed phenytoin and thiamine and a salbutamol inhaler. Two weeks later you are informed that he is brought to hospital by ambulance after suffering a tonic-clonic seizure. What is the most likely aetiology of this?

    a. Fluoxetine has affected plasma levels of phenytoin

    b. Fluoxetine may have reduced the seizure threshold

    c. Hepatic encephalopathy

    d. Erratic use of phenytoin due to a return to alcohol misuse

    e. It could be any of the above

The Case of Ms D

13. Ms D is a 20-year-old university student who presents with low mood of 4 weeks duration. You screen for depressive symptoms and diagnose a mild to moderate depressive episode. She does not like medication. What could you recommend?

    a. Referral for counselling

    b. Self-help and bibliotherapy

    c. Exercise

    d. A balanced diet

    e. Any or all of the above

14. Ms D presents again in 8 weeks and her mood is much worse. She is not eating well, is losing weight and has stopped attending university. She is yet to see a counsellor as the waiting list is lengthy. She agrees to an antidepressant and you prescribe escitalopram. The following week, she returns to your surgery full of energy, is talking continuously and difficult to interrupt. She has not been sleeping and in the consultation, becomes flirtatious. What is the first step in respect of pharmacotherapy?

    a. Commence sodium valproate

    b. Commence melatonin

c. Stop the escitalopram

d. Commence lamotrigine

e. Commence zopiclone

15. Ms D is seen in secondary care and diagnosed with bipolar affective disorder. She recovers from her mood symptoms. You see her 18 months later. She has dropped out of her university course but is in a stable relationship. She has been discharged from secondary care. She is now on no medication. She consults you in respect of medication to prevent relapses in the future. Which of the following are you least likely to recommend?

a. Risperidone

b. Lithium

c. Olanzapine

d. Lamotrigine

e. Sodium valproate

The Case of Mr E

16. Mr E is 83 years old and suffers with dementia. He lives in a nursing home. He has a history of depression 30 years ago but has not been on any medication for over 20 years. He has just returned from hospital after treatment for a myocardial infarction. Staff at the home, with whom he has a good relationship, report that he is becoming more withdrawn, and is tearful. His appetite is poor. You consider prescribing an antidepressant. What would be your preference?

a. Sertraline

b. Escitalopram

c. Amitryptiline

d. Venlafaxine

e. Tranylcypromine

17. You assess Mr E and find that he is moderately depressed. He is not suicidal. You wish to prescribe sertraline. You find that his dementia affects his capacity to make decisions about this and he does not have the capacity to consent to the antidepressant. How would you proceed?

a. Recommend involuntary admission to a psychiatric ward

b. Ask for the antidepressant to be covertly administered in soup

c. Conduct an assessment of his 'best interests' on how to proceed

d. Approach the courts for a decision on how to proceed

e. Prescribe the medication, ignoring the issue around capacity

18. Mr E is prescribed an SSRI in his best interest and recovers from his depressive episode within 8 weeks. However, staff contact you to say that he is more confused and agitated. Which of the following would you consider?

    a. Delirium unrelated to the treatment for depression

    b. Gastrointestinal bleed

    c. Hyponatremia

    d. A vascular event

    e. It could be any of the above

The Case of Mr F

19. Mr F is a 24-year-old librarian who has become reluctant to leave the house over the last 6 months. He becomes anxious at the thought of going out, fearing he will faint or blush and become embarrassed. This is affecting his ability to go to work. What would you recommend in the first instance?

    a. Benzodiazepines

    b. Pregabalin

    c. Phenelzine

    d. Referral to a psychologist for cognitive behavioural therapy (CBT)

    e. Mindfulness

20. Mr F engages in CBT but after 14 sessions, still has troubling symptoms. What is the first step in respect of pharmacotherapy?

    a. Commence phenelzine

    b. Commence propranolol

    c. Commence escitalopram

    d. Commence pregabalin

    e. Commence diazepam

21. Mr F reports at a follow up consultation that he is coping with the anxiety by drinking alcohol. He reports consuming one glass of wine (2 units) a night to help him sleep. What would now be your management plan?

    a. Stop the antidepressant and attempt a brief intervention around alcohol

    b. Continue the antidepressant and attempt a brief intervention around alcohol

    c. Stop the antidepressant and add disulfiram

    d. Continue the antidepressant and add disulfiram

    e. Refer to secondary care

The Case of Ms G

22. Ms G is 31 years old and has always been an anxious person. She works as a domestic cleaner. More recently, she has troubling thoughts that her hands are dirty with germs. She finds these thoughts to be intrusive and hard to resist. They make her anxious. She has begun washing her hands several times a day. She is able to work and manage her home life but would like to get help with these symptoms as she knows that her handwashing is excessive. What would you recommend in the first instance?

    a. Diazepam before a work shift

    b. Low-dose quetiapine

    c. A period of time off work

    d. Referral for brief cognitive behavioural therapy (CBT) – Exposure and Response Prevention

    e. Wearing gloves during work

23. Ms G comes back in a few weeks. She is still on the waiting list for CBT and her symptoms are becoming more problematic. She now wakes up at night just to wash her hands as she fears they are contaminated. She knows this does not make any sense. Her family life is suffering. How would you proceed?

    a. Recommend admission to a psychiatric ward

    b. Commence a hypnotic such as zopiclone at a low dose

    c. Commence an SSRI such as escitalopram and maintain at a low dose

    d. Commence an SSRI such as escitalopram and titrate to a higher dose

    e. Refer to secondary care

24. In what circumstances would you refer Ms G to secondary care for an opinion?

    a. Not responding to adequate trial on SSRI for a period of 3 months on a therapeutic dose

    b. Acute suicidal crisis

    c. Severe and disabling symptoms

    d. If uncertain about the risks associated with intrusive sexual, aggressive, or death-related thoughts

    e. Any of the above

The Case of Miss H

25. Miss H is a 14-year-old girl, who is presenting with low mood, anhedonia, and poor self-esteem. These symptoms have been present for the last 4 weeks and are affecting her performance at school. You diagnose a mild depressive episode. What would you recommend in the first instance?

    a. Escitalopram

    b. Venlafaxine

    c. Short course of benzodiazepines

    d. Cognitive behavioural therapy (CBT)

    e. Risperidone

26. Miss H has completed 8 sessions of CBT. However, there is a worsening in the severity of her depressive symptoms. She now presents with low mood, anhedonia, low energy levels, initial insomnia, poor appetite, and fleeting suicidal ideation. What is the first step in respect of pharmacotherapy?

    a. Escitalopram

    b. Venlafaxine

    c. Fluoxetine

    d. Short course of benzodiazepines

    e. Risperidone

27. Miss H reports she has a fear of taking tablets/capsules and becomes very anxious around the time of swallowing tablets/capsules. What would you recommend in this instance?

    a. Stop fluoxetine and continue CBT only

    b. Watchful waiting

    c. Switch to risperidone oro-dispersible

    d. Switch to IV citalopram

    e. Switch to a liquid preparation of fluoxetine

28. Miss H is currently on maximum dosage of fluoxetine and reports a significant improvement in her depressive symptoms. However, her sleep remains disturbed and is affecting her functioning. What would you recommend?

    a. Short-term risperidone

    b. Short-term diazepam

    c. Short-term melatonin

    d. Long-term zopiclone

    e. Long-term promethazine

The Case of Boy J

29. Boy J is a 10-year-old boy who presents with a 6-month history of impaired concentration, running and jumping excessively and often interrupts other children at school. These symptoms adversely impact his school performance and he is unable to complete his homework. His parents describe him as a bright and intelligent child who can be impulsive. What would be the most likely diagnosis in this case?

    a. Childhood schizophrenia

    b. Anxiety disorder

    c. Hyperkinetic disorder (also commonly known as ADHD)

    d. Selective mutism

    e. Reading disorder

30. What is the male-to-female ratio in community presentations of hyperkinetic disorder?

    a. 4 : 1

    b. 1 : 1

    c. 10 : 1

    d. 1 : 4

    e. 1 : 2

31. Boy J is seen by a specialist and diagnosed with hyperkinetic disorder. What is the first step in respect of the pharmacotherapy?

    a. Benzodiazepines

    b. Pregabalin

    c. Fluoxetine

    d. Olanzapine

    e. Methylphenidate

The Case of Boy K

32. Boy K is a 15-year-old boy who is presenting with excessive hand washing for the last 3 months. This has resulted in dry skin and some bruises on his hands. What would you recommend in first instance?

    a. Watchful waiting

    b. Commence escitalopram

    c. Cognitive behavioural therapy (CBT) with exposure and response prevention

    d. Family therapy

    e. Rational emotive behaviour therapy

33. You wish to objectively assess the severity of obsessive compulsive disorder so that you can monitor the response to treatment. Which of the following scales would you use?

    a. Children's Depression Inventory (CDI)

    b. Social Communication Questionnaire (SCQ)

    c. Children's Yale-Brown Obsessive Compulsive Scale (C-YBOCS)

    d. Positive and Negative Syndrome Scale (PANSS)

    e. Young Mania Rating Scale (YMRS)

34. Boy K has completed 6 sessions of CBT. However, he is finding it very difficult to cope with his symptoms which are impacting his academic performance. Both his parents and Boy K ask for a trial of medication. What would be your first choice of medication?

    a. Sertraline

    b. Paroxetine

    c. Pregabalin

    d. Venlafaxine

    e. Citalopram

35. How long would you continue the pharmacological treatment for Boy K?

    a. 3 months following remission of symptoms

    b. 3 months once titrated to the maximum dosage

    c. No longer than 12 months

    d. No longer than 6 months

    e. 6 months following remission of symptoms

The Case of Mr L

36. Mr L presents to your surgery complaining of restlessness. He has increased activity during the day, marked talkativeness and over-familiarity. His partner confirms that Mr L 'is not himself' and previously had an episode of depression. What is the most likely diagnosis?

    a. Normal mood

    b. Hypomania

    c. Mania with psychotic symptoms

    d. Mania without psychotic symptoms

    e. Agitated depression

37. Careful history-taking reveals that Mr L had an episode of mania with psychotic symptoms in the past, but stopped taking medication. Which medication is optimal for maintenance treatment in bipolar disorder?

    a. Valproate

    b. Lithium

    c. Lamotrigine

    d. Olanzapine

    e. Diazepam

38. Three months after being commenced on lithium by a community mental health team, Mr L presents to your surgery in an agitated state with slurred speech and strange behaviour. What diagnosis do you need to rule out as a matter of urgency?

    a. Mania with psychotic symptoms

    b. Side effects of lithium

    c. Mania without psychotic symptoms

    d. Lithium toxicity

    e. Agitated depression

The Case of Ms M

39. Ms M, a 17-year-old woman, presents to your surgery at the request of her mother. Ms M says her mother is worried because Ms M thinks she is 'fat' and has lost weight by avoiding certain foods. She exercises excessively and no longer has periods. What is the most likely diagnosis?

    a. Bulimia nervosa

    b. Normal weight loss

    c. Anorexia nervosa

    d. Binge eating disorder

    e. Dissociation

40. You suggest referral to specialist mental health services but Ms M is worried. She asks what will be the main kind of treatment she needs. Which is the correct answer to her question?

    a. Antidepressant medication

    b. Psychoanalytic psychotherapy

    c. Cognitive behavioural therapy

    d. Antipsychotic medication

    e. A 'watch and wait' approach

41. Ms M's mother asks to speak with you, and Ms M agrees to this. Ms M's mother asks how quickly Ms M should regain weight. Which is the best approach?

    a. Ms M should gain weight as quickly as possible

    b. Ms M should not gain weight at all

    c. Ms M should gain weight over the course of a year

    d. Ms M should not weigh herself

    e. Weight gain should be steady rather than dramatic

Miscellaneous

42. How is most psychiatric care provided?

    a. In psychiatric hospitals, to involuntary psychiatry patients

    b. In general hospitals, to medically ill patients

    c. In psychiatric hospitals, to voluntary psychiatry patients

    d. Through online mental health portals

    e. By primary care teams and community mental health services

43. Which psychiatric conditions are most commonly associated with involuntary psychiatric care?

    a. Alcohol and substance misuse disorders

    b. Schizophrenia and mood disorders

    c. Personality disorders

    d. Severe obsessive compulsive disorder

    e. Life-threatening eating disorders

44. The initial decision about referral for consideration for involuntary care should be what kind of decision?

    a. Legal

    b. Judicial

    c. Clinical

    d. Custodial

    e. Financial

45. Globally, how many people are estimated to die by suicide each year?

    a. 8 million

    b. 800,000

    c. 100,000

    d. 1,000

    e. 80,000

46. How should you ask someone about their suicidal ideation?

   a. Not at all

   b. In a vague, roundabout way

   c. In an indirect, drawn-out fashion

   d. Through a third party

   e. In a sympathetic, direct, matter-of-fact way

47. What is the most important part of the consultation with someone who has suicidal thoughts?

   a. Phoning their family

   b. Listening

   c. Asking more questions

   d. Requesting tests

   e. Speaking

Self-Assessment Answers

The Case of Mrs A

1. a   2. c   3. d   4. c   5. e

The Case of Ms B

6. b   7. c   8. b   9. b

The Case of Mr C

10. d   11. b   12. e

The Case of Ms D

13. e   14. c   15. e

The Case of Mr E

16. a   17. c   18. e

The Case of Mr F

19. d   20. c   21. b

The Case of Ms G

22. d   23. d   24. e

The Case of Miss H

25. d   26. c   27. e   28. c

The Case of Boy J

29. c   30. a   31. e

The Case of Boy K

32. c   33. c   34. a   35. e

The Case of Mr L

36. b   37. b   38. d

The Case of Ms M

39. c   40. c   41. e

Miscellaneous

42. e   43. b   44. c   45. b   46. e   47. b

Index

Psychiatry Algorithms for Primary Care, First Edition. Gautam Gulati,
Walter Cullen, and Brendan Kelly.
© 2021 John Wiley & Sons Ltd. Published 2021 by John Wiley & Sons Ltd.